GREAT GRUB FOR TODDLERS

Cas Clarke wrote her first book, *Grub on a Grant*, after taking a degree in Urban Studies at Sussex University. She now lives in a rural retreat in Surrey with her husband Andy, toddler James and baby Helena.

Also by Cas Clarke

Grub on a Grant
Feast Your Friends
Peckish but Poor
Mean Beans
Posh Nosh
Vegetarian Grub on a Grant

Great Grub
for Toddlers

Fuss-free Cooking for
Babies and Under-5s

Cas Clarke

HEADLINE

First published in 1998
by HEADLINE BOOK PUBLISHING

10 9 8 7 6 5 4 3 2 1

Illustrations by Mike Gordon

ISBN 0 7472 5662 4

Typeset by
Letterpart Limited, Reigate, Surrey

Printed in England by
Clays Ltd, St Ives plc

HEADLINE BOOK PUBLISHING
A division of Hodder Headline PLC
338 Euston Road
London NW1 3BH

For James and Helena

Contents

Acknowledgements

In my quest to find out just what babies and toddlers really are eating (as opposed to what books tell us they should eat) I have had a great deal of help from various friends and acquaintances. I would, however, particularly like to thank the following: Louise – mother of George, Humphrey and Charles; Lucy – mother of Christian and Guy; Sue – Henry's mother; Wendy – mother of Thomas, Delyth and Joseph; Claire – Brendan's mother; and Sarah – Ben, Oliver and Patrick's mother.

Introduction

Once upon a time there was a world where meat and two vegetables were considered to be the perfect meal for growing children and the children were very lucky if their parents could afford to feed them in such a fashion. Well-behaved children (seen but not heard) were sat down at a table and given virtually the same menus week in and week out.

Okay, a bit of a myth, but still, how life has changed! For the majority of parents the problems of feeding children have changed dramatically. We are now continually bombarded with information – often in much more technical detail than we can usefully assess – about our food and its nutritional value. Although we live in an affluent age, the benefits this wealth brings have been eroded by some of the processes that our foodstuffs have gone through before reaching our tables.

Meateaters have been worried by the BSE scare, and those who have sought a 'healthier' diet and turned to chicken have had to deal with the increasing amount of salmonella found in poultry. Fish was promoted as an ideal 'health' food, but how healthy can a fish from polluted seas be? And it now appears that with fish stocks falling so dramatically, because of the overfishing that has taken place, fish could become increasingly difficult to obtain – unless farmed, and there have been many concerns voiced over the health of farmed fish. Many people have turned to vegetarianism as the answer, only to find that pesticides prevail in many fruit and vegetables. Milk, eggs, cheese, bread – basics of diets of yesteryear – have all had questions raised about their safety/nutritional values over the past years. Where does that leave us?

Unfortunately the answer appears to be up the creek without a paddle!

Having been an avid reader on all aspects of culinary conundrums over the last decade I have come to the conclusion (along with many others I suspect) that there is only so much that we can do to safeguard our health. In order to live we have to ingest food – at least until the perfect pill appears (and if it were available, who would wish to give up the many pleasures of eating? Certainly not me, I very much enjoy the social aspect of eating and drinking). Since we cannot, individually, truly ascertain the safety of our food, we have to waive some of our food fears in order merely to exist.

Of course we have worries about our own health, but what parent does not worry tenfold over the health of their children? Although I will happily feed myself and my husband with dishes containing beef, I cannot feel the same about feeding it to my two children. Unhappily, since the government was so lax in making available accurate information on our beef, there really has been a breakdown in consumer confidence. The only beef my daughter had before she was one year old was that supplied to me by Heal Farm, a farm in Devon that specialises in 'kind' farming and rare/traditional breeds.

In many cases I have changed to using either lamb or venison mince where formerly I would have used beef, as have lots of people as you can see from the different types of mince now commonly found in the shops. For convenience I was willing to believe the meat industry when it said that beef was now safe – when it came to feeding the adults in our family – but I was not willing to risk the children!

As with many aspects of feeding children, there is a lot of emotional baggage to deal with.

I actually believe that it is probably easier to feed our children than we are being told. After all, most people didn't have the perfect diet when they were young and at the end of the day does it really matter? Especially when you consider some of the things that we do to our bodies as we get older! Moderation, as in all things, is probably the best road to take.

Above all, my main aim in feeding our own two children has been to try and ensure that they enjoy their mealtimes. Yes, I have also tried to get them to eat a healthy, balanced diet, but at the end of the day if I have fostered a love of good food and of good company at mealtimes I will be more than happy. (I suppose good table manners would really be the icing on the cake!)

I can outline my philosophy quite simply:

1. There are no hard and fast rules when it comes to feeding children. What will work with one child may not work for another. Do whatever is right for you and your family.

2. Try not to feel guilty if you can't provide delicious, nutritionally balanced meals three times a day, every day! Some childcare books read as if you have a full-time cook, giving examples of menus for cooked breakfasts, lunches, teas, etc. I just don't think that this is physically possible – whatever people tell you!

3. Quite simply make sure that mealtimes are fun, and by this I don't mean that you have to dress the food up to make it appear to be something else. Keep portion sizes small – nothing puts a toddler off faster than a mountain of food on his plate. Ensure that you sit down with your children and eat with them. Chat to your children, make them feel involved with the meal. At some point between two and two and a half they will be able to start helping to lay the table, handing round serving dishes, helping themselves and pouring out drinks! (Very messy at first!) All this appeals to youngsters and will help to get them interested in coming to their meals.

4. Most importantly I would never, ever make a child eat something they didn't want to eat. I am inordinately proud of James whenever he tries something that he thinks he won't like. If he then refuses it that's fine by me – at least by trying it there's hope that he might like it. Every parent knows how heartbreaking it is to cook for your child only for them to take one look and refuse most adamantly to even take a tiny taste! It's this trait, which appears to be universal, that really undermines parents' attempts to feed their children a varied diet.

Throughout the book I have used examples of very real children and what they actually eat, their likes and dislikes. Friends have been kind enough to give me some sample menus so that you can see just how different children's likes and dislikes can be. This book is full of the recipes that we use to feed our own two little monkeys, and I hope it will serve as a practical guide for other busy parents. It recognises that although we aim to give our children a healthy balanced diet, we do at times fall short of this, and that in our modern busy lives we do sometimes have to rely on convenience foods – look at the space that supermarkets devote to fresh produce and the aisles and aisles of convenience foods, then look at what shoppers have in their trolleys and it soon becomes clear that many people rarely 'cook' at all.

I should mention that there is absolutely no rhyme or reason as to how I have used 'him', 'her', 'mum', 'dad' or whether I talk about feeding a single child or the five thousand. I have to admit that when writing I am generally thinking about the last person I cooked that particular recipe for and so if the text refers to someone it will be the person or people I am thinking about at that particular time. I certainly couldn't choose one sex to refer to, as some writers do, or change pronouns in alternate chapters. Similarly if I mention mum I sometimes (if I remember) then add dad in brackets. This is not deriding dad – or grandma, friend, nanny, etc. – it's just that mum was the first word that came to hand. It certainly is not always mum who takes the main responsibility for the family offspring, as you can quickly discover by visiting your local baby and toddler group. So please read whatever you like into titles.

In the following chapters I hope you will find how to fit feeding your little darling into your own lifestyle: it is never easy or hassle free, forget all images you may have of sweetly serene mothers and perfectly behaved, clean children, sitting happily around a table. All you can reasonably hope for is a well-fed child and the (possible) retention of your sanity!

And remember, nobody is perfect and the superparent doesn't exist. (I expect when Lois Lane and Superman produce children we will finally have our proof of this.)

1. Helpful hints

What to expect

At the beginning parents should have no difficulty in deciding how to feed their baby. There is ample information explaining that for newborn infants breast is best. Breast milk is a complete food for the newborn. This doesn't mean that in deciding to breastfeed your baby you will have no problems. Everyone has seen pictures of doting mothers smiling down at their suckling baby. In real life breastfeeding is not always easy. No one had prepared me for the absolute agony of those first few days. The only way I can describe it is that it felt like someone was trying to suck my nipples through a very small straw! It was excruciating. As I surveyed my ragged, bleeding and very sore nipples the temptation to give in and resort to formula milk was extremely strong. However, after three weeks of this agony it did start to get better and thereafter I agree it was much easier to feed James.

The next problem that parents worry about is whether their little darling is actually getting enough to thrive on. This is difficult to believe when they appear to want feeding every hour! And since each feed can take approximately an hour, this means you start to feel as if your sole purpose in life is being a feeding machine. These are desperate hours, and only those who have gone through it can really understand just how low a mother can get at this time. One day you're a free spirit, the next you have ceased to exist as a person, you appear to be there only to serve this tiny little person's every whim and desire. You desperately love this little scrap of humanity *but*, and it is a big but, you are sore, miserable and drop-dead exhausted. I think it is love that keeps you going at this point and hopefully support from your partner. It seems to go on forever and then at last there are little chinks of light. The baby's feeding starts to fall into a pattern, the little darling looks up at you and smiles (and you know it's not wind). The baby sleeps through the night! These are the milestones that so help parents through those first weeks and months. If you're exceedingly lucky you could be through the worst by three months as I was with my second child. James was a tougher nut to crack. It was a year before I began to feel like a human being again. He was a very demanding baby, but it was the five o'clock starts that I found so exhausting with him. Every baby is different, every parent's experience is unique. You will certainly always have a riveting topic of conversation with complete strangers!

More on breastfeeding

The advice with breastfeeding is that once the baby is correctly latched on initial soreness should soon disappear. Feed on one breast until empty and then offer the other breast if the baby still seems hungry. Then on the next feed start on the second breast. It's all very simple in theory, but not quite so easy in practice. For instance, although the midwife always said don't let the baby fall asleep at the breast, you try stopping them! Then when you realise that your little darling is actually asleep and try to remove them to their cot, they wake up screaming and ravenously hungry. Yep, it's back on the breast time. This is why one feed can commonly take an hour.

Even this wouldn't be so bad if the baby then slept for the four hours they supposedly sleep in between feeds – 'You should be so lucky, lucky, lucky, lucky . . .' Although I have known a couple of babies start out this way (who, by coincidence, were born within a couple of weeks of each other) it was only a matter of time before they were running their mothers ragged.

Just for the fun of it, I jotted down some of Helena's feeding patterns that first week. (Might seem like a strange thing to do, but what else is there to do in the wee hours of the morning!) We brought her home on the Sunday lunchtime; she'd been born that morning and mother was dying to get home to have a nap. I had my mother and Andy at home so I knew I had more chance of getting a rest there than at the hospital. It's a well-known fact that nurses, midwives and health visitors always appear the moment you've just succeeded in getting the baby to sleep. So unless you have someone else to help with the baby, rest is absolutely impossible.

She slept a lot the first couple of days both at night and during the day, then the fun started!

The table overleaf shows that babies sleep a lot less than you expect them to! Before embarking on becoming parents we were under this strange impression that babies slept, were fed, had their nappies changed and were only briefly awake before once more going to sleep. What did she do when she was not sleeping or feeding? Crying, looking puzzled, crying, mewing, crying, looking amazed, crying and yes more crying . . .

It also shows that her most active period was between ten o'clock at night and five o'clock in the morning. This lasted for a number of weeks. In fact, although she would sleep in her crib during the day, she absolutely refused to go in it at night, and when you have another small child in an adjoining bedroom you tend to give in to the screaming baby quite quickly rather than risk having them both awake. This did happen a couple of times and at these points our bed seemed to resemble Charing Cross more than the place where we hoped to sleep! She also generally liked attention in the early evening (a very common trait in

Helena's Feeding/Sleeping Pattern

	Tuesday	Wednesday	Thursday	Friday	Saturday
9am–12 noon	slept 2 hours fed 30 minutes	slept 2 hours fed 30 minutes	slept 1 hour fed 25 minutes	slept 2 hours fed 15 minutes	slept 2 hours fed 35 minutes
12 noon–6pm	slept 4 hours fed 30 minutes	slept 3 hours fed 85 minutes	slept 4 hours fed 40 minutes	slept 3 hours fed 45 minutes	slept 4 hours fed 20 minutes
6pm–10pm	slept 1 hour fed 70 minutes	slept 3 hours fed 40 minutes	slept 2 hours fed 40 minutes	slept 15 minutes fed 1 hour	slept 2 hours fed 45 minutes
10pm–5am	slept 1 hour fed 90 minutes	slept 1 hour fed 65 minutes	slept 4 hours fed 50 minutes	slept 5 hours fed 25 minutes	slept 3 hours fed 55 minutes
5am–9am	slept 2 hours fed 30 minutes	slept 3 hours fed 15 minutes	slept 2 hours fed 35 minutes	slept 3 hours fed 30 minutes	slept 2 hours fed 1 hour
Total sleeping time	10 hours	12 hours	13 hours	13 hours 15 minutes	13 hours
Time spent feeding	4 hours 10 minutes	3 hours 55 minutes	3 hours 10 minutes	2 hours 55 minutes	3 hours 35 minutes

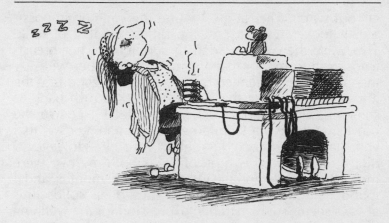

new babies – this was the point of the day when James used to drive us to absolute distraction). I would generally be trying to feed her at about ten o'clock when she had quietened down a little and Andy would nip upstairs for a nap, then around one-thirty to two o'clock, after she had had another little feed, I would pass her over to Andy who would watch some late-night TV with her while mother grabbed a couple of hours' sleep. Then at five o'clock she would normally have a feed and we could both settle down for a couple of hours before it all started again!

We did wonder if this pattern of sleeping was due to the fact that she had been born at night because we hadn't had this problem with James who was born in the daytime. It took four or five weeks before we could turn her around and she started to have her main sleep at night, and then at six weeks old she slept through the night for the first time. Within another couple of weeks she was regularly sleeping through the night and continues to do so unless for a very good reason such as teething or feeling off colour. Bliss!

After you have been breastfeeding for a while you will have to try and express your milk because until you do this you are always tied to the baby, never able to get out without her at all. I found this nigh on impossible; it took forever to get the tiniest amount of milk. This was when we decided to supplement her breastfeeds with formula milk. I can still remember with joy the freedom experienced by being able to get out of the house and knowing that I didn't need to rush back as someone else could give her a bottle! Of course the downside to giving supplemental formula feeds is that you start to produce less milk yourself. However, I didn't really find this a problem as both my two were more than ready for weaning by three months and I found in both cases that once started on solids (this always seems such a strange expression for the weaning foods) both started to be less interested in breast milk. By four months James was only being breastfed early in the morning and late at night and had his last breastfeed the day he was five months. I had intended to breastfeed Helena until she was six months but at three and a half months she was down to just morning and night feeds and gave up completely just before she was four months old.

I had hoped to feed her until she was six months because James developed eczema just as I had given up breastfeeding him and I had been told that if I had fed him to six months this may not have developed – strange how you're never told these snippets of information before the event! However, in the end I went on a diet while I was feeding Helena (a very lax one allowing 1800 calories a day) and within a week my milk had dried up completely. So be warned, don't diet if you intend to carry on breastfeeding.

If, for whatever reason, you decide not to breastfeed at the start then there really appears to be no difference in the many formula milks available. However, think very carefully before opting to take this path as it is virtually impossible to reverse your decision. Even if you were only to feed your baby yourself for a few weeks you would be giving your child the best possible start, for the mother's milk as well as being the perfectly balanced food for your baby, containing all the nutrients he needs, also contains antibodies which help protect your baby against infections. Coupled with this is the fact that it is always ready on demand and is easy for the baby to digest – breastfed babies don't have such smelly poo! Breast milk is also less likely to cause stomach upsets, something you really don't want in a small baby.

So please, please, please breastfeed your baby even if only for a short time (it is an incredible experience, once the initial pain has gone, and one I would have been very sorry to have missed). Conversely, if you do decide for whatever reason not to breastfeed (some women find it extremely difficult, or there is the occasional medical reason which makes it inadvisable) don't feel guilty and don't let anyone put you down. You'll have quite enough to deal with without adding to your pressures. Again this is easy to say in theory but very difficult in practice. Because of the emphasis on breast-feeding nowadays, mothers who do decide to bottle-feed can feel immeasurably guilty, and when your hormones are still running amok it can reduce you to tears to have to give your darling baby a bottle when you really want to breastfeed him. Just hold on to the fact that when you look around you, can you spot the people who were breastfed as children? I know I can't!

The general advice on whether your baby is getting enough milk – which is difficult to judge when you are breastfeeding as you can't tell how much milk the baby is getting or whether he is full or not because unfortunately neither breasts nor babies come with reassuring monitors that tell you when they are full or empty – is that you can be sure that the baby is getting enough by its weight gain. This is why new mothers are so fanatical about getting their babies weighed regularly. Generally babies should feed at least five or six times a day and have plenty of wet nappies. Newborn babies can easily go through eight to ten nappies a day, but this soon reduces to five or six once they are starting to get into a pattern and after a few months will reduce to four or five.

The more your baby suckles at the breast the more milk will be produced; this is why if you start to introduce supplementary bottles your milk supply will start to drop. You will also produce less milk if you don't get some rest and a decent diet. This is really when a supportive partner or mother comes in handy because otherwise it is virtually impossible to cope with feeding a small baby and keeping up with her other needs, i.e. clean clothes and bedding, cuddles and vain attempts to keep her amused and prevent her from crying the house down. (I presume that you have already handed over other chores such as cooking, cleaning and shopping.) A really simple diet is called for at this stage, a cheese sandwich is my own personal standby with a drink of milk and a piece of fruit to follow. Beans on toast is another simple standby as are jacket potatoes or pasta with an easy sauce. However, these don't have the advantage of the sandwich, which can be eaten with one hand while feeding the baby without endangering its health (unless you eat all food cold as a matter of course). Incidentally, never ever drink a hot drink while feeding a baby, their skins are very sensitive and can be scalded easily if you spill it.

Principles of nutrition

The basic principles of nutrition regarding babies and toddlers do vary slightly from adult guidelines and it's because of these slight variations that there have been some instances of youngsters from 'middle-class' homes having mild cases of malnutrition. So it is important to understand the different requirements of babies and young children.

For healthy adults and children of school age it is recommended that very roughly a third of calories consumed come from fruit and vegetables, a third from bread, cereals or potatoes, and the rest being divided between meat, fish or other protein foods, milk and dairy products and small amounts of fatty foods.

For small children, who have a much higher need for energy foods than other groups, it is necessary to increase the amount of fatty foods as these are the most concentrated energy foods and it is only through eating them that a child with a small appetite can gain enough calories to meet their energy requirements. Food items that are particularly unsuitable for young children are low-fat spreads and skimmed or semi-skimmed milk. Unless you have a very overweight child it is recommended that until the age of five children have a pint of full-cream milk (or equivalent in dairy produce) per day. This is to provide enough calories to help fulfil the child's energy requirements and plenty of protein, minerals and vitamins essential to the growing child.

There are some fatty foods, however, that are not recommended. These are saturated fats, the main sources of which are animal fats and foods like cake, biscuits and chocolate. Dairy food contains some saturated fats but compensates by being a good source of calcium and protein.

Sugar is the biggest enemy in children's diets; it has no nutrients and provides only calories (which would be better consumed in a form which also provides essential nutrients). It is also the main cause of tooth decay. So beware of processed foods that contain a lot of sugar and certainly don't add sugar to foods. It can come in many guises so watch out for dextrose, glucose, fructose, sucrose, etc.

If you do allow your children sweets it is better for their teeth if they are consumed as part of a meal. For example, if my children are having chocolate they have it after lunch, and if you can clean their teeth afterwards, even better. And on the subject of tooth decay, do be careful of fizzy drinks. These have been shown to have very detrimental effects on teeth so even if your children are having reduced-sugar varieties ensure that they are limited to being part of a meal and try to ensure that teeth are cleaned after consuming.

Processed foods are generally unsuitable for very small children; most do not contain the high proportion of nutrients required, many contain too much saturated fat and sugar and can often have large amounts of salt added which should not be part of a baby's meal at all. So if your family relies heavily on processed foods, having small children is the perfect excuse to change the family's eating patterns so that everyone has a healthier diet.

In the recipes in this book I have rarely added salt when cooking. If you find this bland you can always add salt to your portion at the table. Some products used do contain salt so not all of the menus are entirely salt free, but the salt content is always kept low.

Food hygiene and safety

When James was a baby I started out by feeding him mainly on jars of commercial baby food. One of my main reasons for this was that I was very worried about preparing foods that then had to be served with sterilised equipment. I was terrified of him having any food poisoning. When they are so small food poisoning is the last thing you want to have to deal with. In the UK there are about forty deaths from food poisoning each year (obviously in 1996 this was considerably higher due to the outbreak of e.coli poisoning in Scotland). One of the groups that is very much at risk is babies and small children, mainly because their resistance to bugs is low and also because the symptoms – vomiting and diarrhoea – lead to dehydration very quickly in small infants which can be fatal. However, following a few simple rules should ensure the safety of your children very easily. Obviously whenever making up any milk feeds all equipment should be sterilised according to the manufacturer's directions. Limit the time that you allow a milk feed to hang around, especially in hot weather – if your baby isn't interested, don't offer the same feed at a later time, always offer a fresh bottle. After twenty-four hours any made-up feed that has not been used should be thrown away and a fresh batch made. I found that when we were unsure of how much Helena would want at any given feed it was easier to sterilise a container and make the milk in this. We then kept it in the fridge and could offer her small amounts, then top it up if she still wanted more.

If you are preparing fresh food on a daily basis normal food hygiene should be quite sufficient. Keep raw food apart from cooked food so that cross contamination does not occur and never undercook food. Make sure that pets are not allowed on any surfaces where food preparation takes place, that hands are washed after visiting the toilet – and after blowing your nose! Also make sure that utensils are kept scrupulously clean and be very careful with liquidisers and food processors, making sure that the blades are thoroughly cleaned. I felt much safer preparing Helena's food because we had a dishwasher which washes with water at a much higher temperature than water used when washing dishes by hand. If you do use a tea towel to dry utensils do ensure that it is changed at least on a daily basis – these can be breeding grounds for germs.

The main problems with food hygiene and safety occur when cooked food is stored and then reheated, so this is where extra care must be taken. Whether you are storing leftovers from commercially prepared or home-made food, certain precautions must be followed. It is recommended that once opened or prepared, food is not left longer than forty-eight hours before being discarded. I have to say that this is something I religiously follow. It is also very important when reheating food that it is cooked thoroughly. I know it is very tempting when you have a bawling baby only to heat the food to the temperature that your baby likes to eat it. To be safe, however, food should be thoroughly cooked through and then left to cool, until at a temperature the baby can eat it.

The main thing to remember is that food can smell and taste fine and yet still poison you, so always keep within the use by date that is marked on the packaging. Bacteria are nearly always present in food and since they multiply exceedingly quickly they can be present in harmful numbers in a short time. Don't forget that liquids can be dangerous too; pasteurised fruit juices may have a long shelf life but once opened must be used up within a few days. If products appear to be thicker or runnier than you expect or seem to have unexpected air bubbles in them, be very cautious. Some products that are contaminated have a slight metallic taste to them. If in any doubt play safe and throw it out. Better to be safe than sorry!

Kitchen gadgets and gismos

How did our grandparents manage! With all the kitchen gadgets now on sale, it can be difficult to decide what will be really useful and what is really a waste of space. The following items are the ones that I have found to be either essential or really useful.

- Plastic bowls and spoons (must be able to be sterilised).

- Feeding cups (travelling ones are the most useful).

- Sterilising system – we opted for a microwave system as we have found that this suited our needs. However, there were two drawbacks. Firstly, it is possible to get caught out by power cuts! Secondly, what do you do when travelling? There used to be a product on sale (like a large plastic drawstring bag) that you put the items to be sterilised into, added tap water, and then half an hour later your items were sterilised. But when we were travelling we had one that sprung a leak. Luckily we were alerted by the drip drip drip otherwise we would have had a disaster, after all sterilising solution is in essence a bleach. Maybe other people had the same problem because it doesn't seem to be on sale any more! So when we travelled with Helena as a small baby, we relied on a plastic box and sterilising tablets.

- Baby bottles and bottle brush.

- Mouli grater (Lakeland Plastics do one that comes with different sized graters; useful when encouraging your child to eat bigger pieces of food).

- Blender – I already had a food processor and was able to order an attachment which is suitable for blending very small amounts of food (can also be used for making breadcrumbs and grinding coffee beans). It came with four glass jars with tops that are very useful for storing food.

I haven't bought anything else specifically for the babies, I've just used normal equipment found in most kitchens, i.e. grater, freezer, microwave oven, ice cube maker, etc., etc. Sorry! I've just remembered something we did buy for Helena but could have done without – a bottle warmer! I had seen friends use them, and although since we had bought it we used it, I never found it any better or quicker to use than the Pyrex jug filled with hot water that we used to warm bottles for James. A classic case of money not well spent!

The stock cupboard

There are days when things don't work out as planned and maybe a trip to the shops never materialises. It does pay to have some basics in the house that you know your child will eat. Obviously for very small babies if you are not breastfeeding it is imperative that you keep a stock of your chosen baby milk powder and I would suggest a carton or two of that same brand in its made-up form. Otherwise the day will come when you haven't had a chance to make the milk yet, the baby has had the last feed that you made up and you can't boil the kettle because there's a power cut. It happens, it really does – babies (especially newborns) attract chaos! For just weaned babies keep some home-made baby food in the freezer or some jars of commercial baby food – just for emergencies. For those who are finger feeding, try and always have some rice or pasta in the cupboard, some cheese in the fridge and some peas or tinned sweetcorn in the cupboard – these ingredients make child-friendly emergency meals. Baked beans and bread are also great standbys and ice-cream in the freezer or yoghurts in the fridge will help you to get by.

Example menus

It's very interesting looking at these menus overleaf and talking to mums about just what they feed their children. It now seems to be very rare to have cooked desserts – flavoured yoghurts and fromage frais win hands down every time as favourites for dessert. These are followed very closely by fruit in its many forms, with apples, grapes and bananas being at the top of the list. Ice-cream in its many forms is also very popular (and is sometimes given as a reward for eating all of the savoury part of the meal).

There are certain vegetables which also appear time and time again. These are sweetcorn and peas, carrots, tomatoes (either as part of a salad or on their own), broccoli, baked beans and green beans. For some reason these seem to be fairly universally popular with children in this age group. Since these vegetables are all quick and easy to prepare this made me wonder if we subconsciously affect our children's choices – are these the vegetables we most often offer them or is there something inherent in these particular vegetables that makes them attractive to children's tastes? It doesn't really matter because if your child will eat most or all of these vegetables they are getting a good and varied selection already.

The most popular cereal is definitely hot oat cereal, again a choice that is popular with mums! Starchy foods are popular with children; bread in its many forms appears again and again, as do pasta and potatoes (particularly jacket potatoes). Rice is not quite as popular but still features on most children's menus.

Meats seem to be equally popular and surprisingly fish is just as popular when it arrives coated in breadcrumbs (or is it the tomato ketchup that often accompanies this and is also universally popular with children?).

On reflection it's a shame that most pubs and restaurants that offer children's fare don't reflect the menus that our children eat at home – perhaps tasty casseroles, shepherd's pie or healthy pasta dishes would be better received than those who only offer burger, sausages or one stodgy pasta dish would expect. And why are chips the ubiquitous accompaniment? Children go through phases with chips and they are not always the child's first choice.

Some caterers are gradually catching on to the fact that children's tastes are more sophisticated than they thought, and wouldn't it be better to offer more healthy alternatives if we want our children to grow up following a healthy diet? We can only wait and see what improvements will follow in this area in the future as the trend in families eating out together grows.

Menu 1
Helena – six months

See charts on following pages.

Although most of the food was puréed or mashed at each meal, I did give her something to gnaw on and pick up with her fingers, for example pieces of broccoli or carrot, assorted slices of fruit, grated cheese, rusk or little baby bread sticks. This served to deflect her attention so that a parent could actually spoonfeed her.

Menu 2
James – two and a half years
Helena – nine months

See charts on following pages.

Menu 3
James – two years nine months
Helena – nearly one year

See charts on following pages.

Menus 2 and 3 were winter menus. In menu 2 I was still blending Helena's food a little and adding a little chopped food to it; by menu 3 I was still chopping up her meat or fish but she was picking up the rest either with her fingers or occasionally her spoon. She was of

Example Menu – Menu 1

	Saturday	Sunday	Monday	Tuesday	Wednesday	Thursday	Friday
Breakfast	Baby muesli and apple purée	Orange juice and rusk	Wheat biscuit and banana	As Saturday	Baby cereal and pear purée	As Sunday	As Monday
Lunch	Avocado and fingers of pizza	Lamb, broccoli and potato	Leek, courgette, baby rice and cheese	Cod, courgette and baby rice	Chicken, carrot and potato	Vegetable sauce with pasta and cheese	Sole, peas and baby rice
	Juice	Juice	Juice	Juice	Juice	Juice	Juice
	Banana, apple, orange juice, custard	Baby yoghurt	Strawberries and cream	Baby yoghurt	Banana and custard	Apple and pear cream	Baby yoghurt
Tea	Broccoli with baby rice and cheese	Banana	Cheese sandwich	Cauliflower with baby rice and cheese	Milky rusk	Cheese sandwich	Banana
	Milk	Milk	Milk	Milk	Milk	Milk	Milk
	Baby yoghurt or fromage frais	Baby yoghurt or fromage frais	Baby yoghurt or fromage frais	Baby yoghurt or fromage frais	Baby yoghurt or fromage frais	Baby yoghurt or fromage frais	Baby yoghurt or fromage frais

Example Menu – Menu 2

	Saturday	Sunday	Monday	Tuesday	Wednesday	Thursday	Friday
Breakfast	Hot oat cereal	Wheat biscuits	Wheat biscuits	Muesli	Hot oat cereal	Muesli	Hot oat cereal
	Juice and toast	Juice and toast	Juice and toast	Juice and toast	Juice and toast	Juice and toast	Juice and toast
Lunch	Baked potatoes with cheese and corn	Chicken, potatoes and broccoli	Leftovers	Pasta with vegetable sauce and cheese	Meatballs with rice and peas	Lamb casserole with rice and carrots	Fish with rice and carrots
	Juice	Juice	Juice	Juice	Juice	Juice	Juice
	Yoghurt and/or fruit	Yoghurt and/or fruit	Yoghurt and/or fruit	Yoghurt and/or fruit	Yoghurt and/or fruit	Yoghurt and/or fruit	Yoghurt and/or fruit
Tea	Soup and a roll	Cheese sandwich	Paste sandwich	Soup and a roll	Cheese sandwich	Paste sandwich	Soup and a roll
	Milk	Milk	Milk	Milk	Milk	Milk	Milk
	Yoghurt and/or fruit	Yoghurt and/or fruit	Yoghurt and/or fruit	Yoghurt and/or fruit	Yoghurt and/or fruit	Yoghurt and/or fruit	Yoghurt and/or fruit

Example Menu – Menu 3

	Saturday	Sunday	Monday	Tuesday	Wednesday	Thursday	Friday
Breakfast	Porridge	Porridge	Wheat biscuit	Hot oat cereal	Hot oat cereal	Wheat biscuit	Hot oat cereal
	Juice and toast	Juice and toast	Juice and toast	Juice and toast	Juice and toast	Juice and toast	Juice and toast
Lunch	Baked potatoes with cheese, salad and corn	Pot roast with potatoes, broccoli and carrots	Lamb casserole with rice, carrots and broccoli	Spag bol with carrots and peas	Chicken casserole with potatoes, peas and cobcorn	Lamb mince with pasta, carrots and peas	Fish casserole with rice, carrots and cobcorn
	Juice	Juice	Juice	Juice	Juice	Juice	Juice
	Ice-cream	Fruit crumble with custard	Fruit crumble with custard	Ice-cream	Bananas with custard	Fruit salad and custard	Ice-cream
Tea	Toasted cheese	Soup and a roll	Soup and a roll	Paste sandwich	Cheese sandwich	Baked beans and fishcake	Baked beans on toast
	Milk	Milk	Milk	Milk	Milk	Milk	Milk
	Yoghurt and/or fruit	Yoghurt and/or fruit	Yoghurt and/or fruit	Yoghurt and/or fruit	Yoghurt and/or fruit	Yoghurt and/or fruit	Yoghurt and/or fruit

course having a pint of 'follow-on' milk daily and some diluted fruit juices, while James also had two milk drinks a day as well as his juices. (In between meals if he is thirsty he has diluted low-sugar lemon squash.) Occasional snacks were also given such as chocolate buttons immediately after lunch, extra fruit, plain biscuits or some Hula Hoops.

Another point to make is that neither of my two eat eggs or cottage cheese. Otherwise I would certainly have included eggs, either hard boiled or scrambled, in my breakfast and tea menus and I would have given them cottage cheese at teatime. If you are confident of your source of eggs you can also include soft-boiled eggs with toast soldiers, but this is unwise with very young children because of the risk of salmonella poisoning (how times have changed!).

Menu 4

Ben – six years
Oliver – four years
Patrick – twenty months

See charts on following pages.

Sandwich fillings vary with children, but favourites are cheese, Dairylea, jam, peanut butter and ham. Snacks can include fruit, plain crisps or Hula Hoops, plain biscuits, and special treats at the weekend may

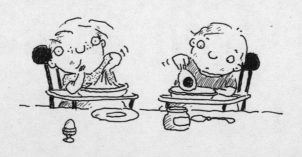

Example Menu – Menu 4

	Saturday	Sunday	Monday	Tuesday	Wednesday	Thursday	Friday
Breakfast	Yoghurt and croissant Fruit juice	Yoghurt and croissant Fruit juice	Cereal and toast Fruit juice	Cereal and toast Fruit juice	Cereal and toast Fruit juice	Cereal and toast Fruit juice	Cereal and toast Fruit juice
Lunch	Pizza and salad	French bread with cheese and tomatoes	Sandwich	Crackers with cheese and salad	Sandwich	Sandwich	Sandwich
	Yoghurt Fruit Fruit juice	Yoghurt Fruit Fruit juice	Yoghurt Fruit Fruit juice	Yoghurt Fruit Fruit juice	Yoghurt Fruit Fruit juice	Yoghurt Fruit Fruit juice	Yoghurt Fruit Fruit juice
Dinner	Grandma's lamb stew with baked potatoes	Pot-roast beef with Yorkshire pudding, roast potatoes, broccoli and carrots	Cod fishcakes, pasta with tomato sauce and peas	Chicken drumsticks with baked potato, carrots and corn	Shepherd's pie with broccoli and corn	Mild chicken curry, rice and peas	Sausages in a bun
	Fruit and/or ice-cream	Fruit and/or ice-cream	Fruit and/or ice-cream	Fruit and/or ice-cream	Fruit and/or ice-cream	Fruit and/or ice-cream	Fruit and/or ice-cream

include gateau perhaps for dessert. If there is any cake in the house, i.e. birthday cake, this is given as dessert. Drink at teatime may be fruit juice, milk or coke depending on circumstances of meal.

Menu 5

George – two years eight months
Humphrey – eighteen months

See charts on following pages
   Drinks are water at home, milk on rising and just before bed. Snacks include biscuits when visiting friends or at toddler groups; sweets are kept as weekend treats (and I think, as in our household, the weekend begins on Friday!). Sandwich fillings include cheese, ham and corned beef (with tomatoes).

Menu 6 (vegetarian and fish)

Brendan – four years

See charts on following pages.
   Snacks mid-morning are either apple or grapes and milk, and mid afternoon a milkshake and occasionally a packet of Hula Hoops. Drinks are apple juice or summer fruit squash with meals.

Example Menu – Menu 5

	Saturday	Sunday	Monday	Tuesday	Wednesday	Thursday	Friday
Breakfast	Boiled eggs and fingers	Bacon, egg and fried bread	Cereal and toast	Cereal and toast	Cereal and toast	Cereal and toast	Cereal and toast
	Orange juice	Orange juice	Orange juice	Orange juice	Orange juice	Orange juice	Orange juice
Lunch	Ham salad	Roast lamb, potatoes and seasonal vegetables	Sandwich and fruit or cheese and apple	Sandwich and fruit or cheese and apple	Sandwich and fruit or cheese and apple	Sandwich and fruit or cheese and apple	Sandwich and fruit or cheese and apple
Dinner	Chops with seasonal vegetables	Fish fingers	Roast chicken with vegetables	Baked potato and baked beans	Meatballs and rice	Pasta and cheese sauce	Casserole with green beans
	Jelly	Yoghurt	Yoghurt or fruit	Yoghurt or fruit	Yoghurt or fruit	Yoghurt or fruit	Yoghurt or fruit

Example Menu – Menu 6

	Saturday	Sunday	Monday	Tuesday	Wednesday	Thursday	Friday
Breakfast	Jam on bread	Jam on bread	Hot oat cereal with raisins	Hot oat cereal with raisins	Hot oat cereal with raisins	Hot oat cereal with raisins	Hot oat cereal with raisins
	Milk	Milk	Milk	Milk	Milk	Milk	Milk
Lunch	Scrambled egg and bread	Chips*	Cottage cheese and bread	Peanut butter sandwich	Emmental and cucumber sandwich	Fried egg sandwich	Peanut butter sandwich
	Yoghurt	Doughnut Coke	Fromage frais	Yoghurt	Yoghurt	Yoghurt	Fromage frais
Dinner	Pizza and salad	Salmon steaks with rice, peas, corn and carrots	Beanburger with pasta, peas and corn	Soya mince with pasta and salad	Fish in breadcrumbs with rice, peas and corn	Quorn in peanut butter, pasta and salad	Lentil bake with pasta, peas, corn and carrots
	Choc-ice	Banana and ice-cream	Cake	Choc-ice	Satsuma and grapes	Cake	Grapes and ice-cream

*This is at the local swimming pool.

2. Weaning

The current advice on weaning is that you shouldn't start to wean your baby on to 'solids' until the baby has reached four months old. You are also advised not to leave it later than six months. The reasoning behind this advice is that most babies' digestive systems are too immature for solids before four months and you increase the risk of allergic reactions. At six months the baby needs more iron and other nutrients than can be provided by milk alone – and if weaning is delayed you will probably incur more resistance when you do start.

However, some babies do seem to be ready for weaning earlier than others and certainly in the past babies were weaned much earlier than this, in some cases virtually from birth! So if you have a screaming infant and you have already tried increasing the milk feeds, check with your health visitor and they will probably advise you to go ahead and start to wean.

I have to admit that I did wean both of mine before they were four months old. I first tried James on baby rice at eleven weeks old – and he wasn't content with just a teaspoonful, from the beginning he had two tablespoons! He really was a hungry baby and soon podged out! After a week I started to give him other flavours and after that there was no looking back – except that when he realised there were better things on offer than plain rice he absolutely refused baby rice after that! I thought that we were going to have to wean Helena even earlier. At nine weeks old she was showing all the signs, chomping anything that came near her mouth, long bouts of crying and generally driving her parents completely round the bend. However, when we did give in and offer some baby rice she completely refused it (who can blame them – it does taste absolutely awful!). It was only a few days since we had changed from 'gold' formula milk to the 'white' for her supplementary bottles and I now believe that she was still getting used to this, because over the next few days the milk did the trick and she settled down again. Helena then went on until fourteen weeks before starting to show signs that she was hungry all the time. This time I tried her on strawberry and apple flavoured baby rice and she loved it, and from then on we were up and running!

Babies are always started on milks that are whey based as their protein is closer to that of breast milk. If your baby appears to be unsatisfied with her feeds you can change to a casein-based milk which helps to make baby feel more full after her feeds and is advertised as being for hungry babies. Then at six months it is best to swap to a 'follow-on' milk as these have a higher iron content which babies of this age need. This should be continued until reaching her first birthday. The manufacturers of these milks recommend that you continue with them until the child's second birthday, but unless you are very worried about your child's diet – particularly whether she is getting enough iron – then I don't feel that the average child really benefits from them after the age of one. And it is great when you can just get the milk out of the fridge rather than have to make it up on a daily basis. The first time I could enter a coffee shop and ask for a milk for Helena was bliss.

Very premature babies and those who are allergic to milk have specialised milks which are prescribed especially for them. If you have a history of allergies in your family it is best to introduce only one new food at a time and wait a couple of days before trying another, this way you will soon learn if there are any foods which upset your baby. Otherwise you can mix flavours to suit you and your child.

You really cannot give a definitive guide as to portion sizes for small children, even in toddlerhood there are enormous differences between them. But during weaning you really don't have to worry as the point is not to start feeding them up but to get them used to the idea of eating solid food and introduce them to as many different flavours as possible. The main source of their nutrition should still be their breastfeeds or at least one pint (20 fl oz or 500ml) of baby milk.

It is always recommended that you start weaning at a time when both you and the baby are feeling relaxed. In reality this is unlikely to happen as the reason you are probably trying to wean your baby is because she is still unsatisfied after her milk feed and so is unlikely to be very happy! It is best to have given her a small breastfeed or bottle before you start or otherwise she will be frantic with hunger. Start with one to two tablespoons and don't expect too much at the beginning. Try at one feed initially and when she is accepting a small amount then start offering food at another feed, building this up to three or four feeds a day. It took Helena a week to get up to three tablespoons of strawberry and apple rice at one meal. I then started her on two meals a day, and after a couple of days started offering small amounts of fruit or vegetable purées at one meal while sticking with the baby rice at breakfast. It was at this point that she was becoming less interested in her breastfeeds so I only breastfed her first thing in the morning and last thing at night, giving her formula feeds during the daytime.

Then when we reached the stage when I gave her banana I started to vary breakfast, alternating between baby rice and fruit purées. It was also at this stage that I started her on three meals a day (she was seventeen weeks old – coincidentally the age I was supposed to have just started weaning her!) and I gave up breastfeeding her as she was completely uninterested. A couple of weeks after this we cut her down to four milk feeds a day and it was at this point that she got into a regular routine of mealtimes that fitted in with the rest of the family. She was then having a milk feed on waking, then breakfast with the family, a milk feed at about half past ten, lunch at twelve o'clock, a milk feed about half past three and tea at five o'clock, with her last bottle just before going to bed at seven o'clock.

To start with the food should be absolutely smooth and very runny and it is probably best to start with something that is similar to milk. This is why most people start with baby rice, although I believe that some people do start with fruit or vegetable purées. Then as your baby gets used to the idea of the food in her mouth and starts to chew you can very gradually add some texture to her meals. This, however, must be a very gradual process and for the first few weeks a very smooth purée is the best route to easy meals. Then you can start to add mashed foods as opposed to blended and then actually start adding chopped food. I did this by blending most of her meal but keeping a little back and finely chopping this before mixing it in. Then you can gradually decrease the amount you blend until finally you can just chop up her meal. Then when it comes to the point when she wants to feed herself, leave her food in pieces that she can easily hold and chew on.

By the time Helena was ten months old she was virtually feeding herself with mummy or daddy occasionally popping a spoonful in for her – this made mealtimes a lot easier. By the way, I am a strong believer in family meals, therefore mother always sits down and eats lunch with her children – in our family the main meal is always at lunchtime. Some people do prefer their children to have their main meal at teatime, and for some children this may help them to sleep through the night. But my two have always been very good at sleeping through and I prefer them to have a good lunch as this will be their routine in their early school years and I think that the less disruption to their routines the better!

The following recipes are the ones that I weaned Helena on and she heartily approved of them all! They appear in the order that I introduced them to Helena.

Recipes

Try your baby with one to two tablespoons initially. Keep a little back for the following meal and using an ice-cube tray freeze the rest. Then when frozen, store the ice-cubes in a clearly labelled freezer bag. This procedure can be followed for all the weaning recipes (except for banana and avocado) thus giving you a stock of ready-made meals for your baby. Then take out the ice-cubes as you need them (defrosting two or three ice-cubes at first and then more as your baby's appetite increases). Either defrost overnight in the fridge or leave at room temperature for one or two hours to defrost. The food can either be thoroughly heated in a micro-wave or in a small saucepan (stirring well) then allowed to cool to the temperature your baby likes and served.

Apple

1 dessert apple

Peel and core the apple, cut into eight segments and put in a small saucepan with enough water to cover. Bring to the boil and then simmer gently for 10–12 minutes or until apple is very soft. Using some of the cooking water, blend until very smooth.

Squash

    1 small butternut squash

Cut in half and remove seeds and pith. Peel and cut the squash into cubes. Put into the top of a steamer and steam until very tender (about 10–12 minutes). Blend until smooth. The flesh is very watery so extra water should not be needed but if you wish you can add a little cooled boiled water.

Squash and apple

This was an all-time favourite with Helena. I got the idea from looking at the range of baby foods produced by Organix whose jars of baby food I always found to be very good standbys – they use only organic ingredients, no emulsifiers, artificial sweeteners or flavourings, or excess water.

    1 small butternut squash
    1 dessert apple

    or
    2 squash ice-cubes
    1 apple ice-cube

Prepare the squash and apple as in the previous recipes and then mix 2 dessertspoons of the squash with 1 dessertspoon of apple. Or defrost ice-cubes and mix together when heating.

Carrot

    1 medium carrot

Peel the carrot and slice thinly, place in a small saucepan and just cover with water. Bring to the boil and then simmer for 10–12 minutes until soft. Blend using some of the cooking water to a smooth purée.

Swede

1 small swede

Peel and cut into cubes, place in a small saucepan and just cover with water. Bring to the boil and then simmer for 20–25 minutes until soft. Blend using just enough of the cooking liquid to produce a smooth purée.

Carrot and swede

I found that Helena also liked mixtures of carrot and apple and swede and apple.

1 medium carrot
1 small swede

or
2 carrot ice-cubes
2 swede ice-cubes

Cook the vegetables as above and then mix 1–2 tablespoons of carrot with an equal amount of swede. Or when heating ice-cubes mix together.

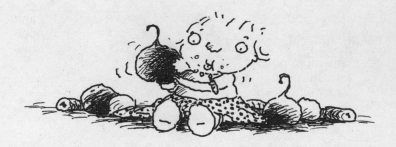

Potato

1 medium potato

Peel potato and cut into cubes. Put into a small saucepan and just cover with water. Bring to the boil and then simmer until soft (about 10–20 minutes). Blend with some of the cooking liquid to a smooth purée.

Parsnip

Helena isn't a big fan of parsnip. I tried her with potato and parsnip but she wasn't too keen on that either, so we didn't bother with parsnips again until we got her onto casseroles – and even then I don't add very much. When she reached the finger food stage we tried her on roast parsnips, but she thought that was yuk! As James also dislikes parsnips we've virtually given them up for the duration.

1 large parsnip

Peel and cut into cubes. Put into a small saucepan and just cover with water. Bring to the boil and then simmer until soft (about 15–20 minutes). Blend with some of the cooking liquid to a smooth purée.

Broccoli

1 small broccoli head

Divide broccoli into florets, place in a small saucepan and just cover with water. Bring to the boil and simmer for 10–15 minutes until soft. Blend using some of the cooking liquid to make a smooth purée.

Potato, broccoli and carrot

1 medium potato
1 small broccoli head
1 medium carrot

or
1 potato ice-cube
1 broccoli ice-cube
2 carrot ice-cubes

Prepare the vegetables as in previous recipes and then mix 1 dessertspoon of potato with an equal amount of broccoli and 2 dessertspoons of carrot. If using ice-cubes mix together when heating.

Banana

It was at this stage that I first introduced Helena to banana – she loved it instantly and became known for a short while as 'Banana Girl' as somehow she always seemed to get it everywhere! By the way, you cannot leave banana in the fridge or it will turn black, but we never had any leftovers as we are all big fans of bananas and I usually buy the small ones anyway as I find that they have a sweeter flavour.

Once your little one will eat banana, life becomes much easier as it is a very nutritious fruit and readily available in many shops and restaurants, so it does make it easier to get out and about. It's the first sign that one day life will return to normal and you won't always have to prepare as for an expedition even for a quick visit to the shops!

1 small banana

Peel and mash the banana until almost liquidy.

Courgette

1 medium courgette

Leave the skin on the courgette, remove the ends and then chop the courgette into small cubes, place in a small saucepan and just cover with water. Bring to the boil and simmer for 5–6 minutes. Alternatively the courgette can be put into the top of a steamer and cooked for 15 minutes, until very soft. Blend into a purée. As courgette is very watery you shouldn't need any extra liquid but use a little of the cooking liquid if you prefer.

Potato, courgette and pea

At this early age I prefer not to give babies a meal of just peas because they are very fibrous. As the baby's digestive system is still very immature I think it's a bit too much to give them anything too fibrous right at the start. This is a nice mixture to introduce them to peas.

> 1 medium potato
> 1 medium courgette
> 2 tablespoons frozen peas

Cook the potato and courgette as in the recipes above but add the peas to the courgette and cook for 5–6 minutes. Blend all three vegetables together into a purée, adding a little of the cooking liquid.

Sweet potato

> 1 medium sweet potato

Peel the sweet potato and cut into cubes, place in a small saucepan and just cover with water. Cook until tender (about 20–30 minutes). Liquidise using just enough of the cooking liquid to produce a smooth purée.

Cauliflower

> 1 small cauliflower head

Divide the cauliflower into florets and place in a small saucepan. Just cover with water and bring to the boil. Simmer for 10–15 minutes. Blend using just enough of the cooking liquid to produce a smooth purée.

Sweet potato and cauliflower

Other good mixtures using cauliflower are broccoli, cauli-flower and carrot and cauliflower and courgette

    1 medium sweet potato
    1 small cauliflower head

    or
    2 sweet potato ice-cubes
    2 cauliflower ice-cubes

Cook the vegetables as in previous recipes and then mix 1–2 tablespoons of the sweet potato with an equal amount of the cauliflower. If using ice-cubes, mix together when heating.

Pear

This was a huge hit with Helena and added a new ingredient to our range of breakfast choices. It can also be used to make another popular choice, pears and apple.

    1 pear

Peel and core the pear, slice and put in a small saucepan with just enough water to cover. Bring to the boil and then simmer until soft (about 8–10 minutes). Liquidise using a little of the cooking liquid if needed to produce a smooth purée.

Papaya

Try also mixing this with pear to make papaya and pear. I also found that Helena particularly liked this mixture with some baby rice to give a slightly thicker texture. (And as papaya is one of the more expensive fruits this makes it go further.)

    1 medium papaya

Cut the fruit in half and remove all of the black seeds. Scoop out all the flesh into the top of a steamer. Steam for 5–6 minutes until soft. This fruit blends very easily so needs no additional liquid.

Avocado

In many parts of the world avocado is used as the main ingredient to wean babies, mainly because it doesn't need cooking, is cheap and in plentiful supply. For us it is not so convenient as, like bananas, it doesn't keep well and it cannot be frozen. However, it is a very nutritious fruit so if you want to give your baby avocado do so at a time when you can use the rest as a lunchtime dish – for instance as part of a salad.

> 1 avocado – soft but not so overripe it is starting to go black

Cut in half and remove the stone. Scoop out ¼–½ of the flesh and mash right down. Use immediately.

With all of these first weaning foods once the baby is adjusting to the idea of solid food you can then start to vary the texture by giving a thicker purée (when you make them up don't add as much or any cooking liquid). You can also start to bulk them out by adding a little plain baby rice which, although very unpopular if given straight, is generally happily accepted when mixed with a flavour that the baby likes. By the way, don't be fooled by a baby's immediate reaction to any flavour. Helena always made a face whenever she had that first spoonful, but then the mouth would open and she would lean forward, as if she thought she had better check again as nothing could really taste that bad!

These recipes should serve you through the first month or two. Then at about five months I like to really start introducing the flavours that we use a lot in our house – after all, the sooner they get used to these the sooner they can eat the same meal as the rest of the family. Also, as your baby's digestive system is getting used to food, you can now add some more fibrous vegetables – but initially they must be put through a sieve or mouli after being puréed as the baby's digestive system still cannot deal with the skins. So be prepared for a lot of wastage when ingredients such as peas, mangetout or green beans are prepared.

We were lucky in this respect because we live very close to a really good P-Y-O farm and these summer crops were available at just the right time for us to use them for Helena, so it didn't cost us a fortune to feed her these lovely vegetables.

Mangetout

200–250g (8–10 oz) mangetout

Top and tail and place in a medium saucepan, just cover with water and bring to the boil. Simmer for 10–12 minutes until soft. Drain and purée and then either put through a mouli or a sieve. Using 2 tablespoons of the resulting smooth purée, mix with some plain baby rice to a consistency that your baby will like.

Fresh peas

200–250g (8–10 oz) peapods

First pop open the peapods and take out the peas. Put the peas in a small saucepan and cover with water. Bring to the boil and simmer for about 10 minutes until tender. Purée and put through a mouli or sieve. Again Helena particularly liked this mixture with some baby rice.

Potato, peas and carrot

1 medium potato
200–250g (8–10 oz) peapods
1 medium carrot

or
2 potato ice-cubes
1 pea ice-cube
1–2 carrot ice-cubes (depending on baby's appetite)

Prepare vegetables as in previous recipes, then mix 2 dessertspoons of potato with 1 dessertspoon of pea and 1–2 dessertspoons of carrot. If using ice-cubes, mix together when heating.

Green beans

200–250g (8–10 oz) green beans

Top and tail the beans and slice diagonally (unless using small beans which can be left whole). Place in a large saucepan and cover with water. Bring to the boil and simmer until soft (10–15 minutes). Purée with a little of the cooking liquid and then put through a mouli or sieve.

Asparagus

Asparagus was and still is a big hit with Helena – obviously a girl with expensive tastes!

100g (4 oz) asparagus

Cut off any wooden ends and then place in the top of a steamer and cook until tender (about 4–8 minutes depending on thickness). Purée and put through a mouli or sieve. As this is an expensive vegetable it should definitely be mixed with baby rice to make it go further.

Tomato

Favourites using tomatoes were mangetout, tomato and carrot; courgette, cauliflower and tomato; and broccoli, tomato and carrot.

4–6 tomatoes

Make a cut in each tomato and then place in boiling water for 1–2 minutes. Drain and remove the skins. Deseed and core, chop the flesh and cook for 2 minutes with a teaspoonful of butter in a small saucepan. Purée. I froze this in an ice-cube tray and used it when making up mixtures for Helena.

Red pepper

Since this is rather a spicy purée when I made up combinations with it I never put more than one pepper ice-cube in a mixture. Green bean, cauliflower and pepper was well received, as was pea, tomato, carrot and pepper.

1 red pepper

Cut in half and remove the seeds and core. Cut the pepper into strips and place in a saucepan. Cover with water, bring to the boil and then simmer for 8–10 minutes until soft. Purée and then put through a mouli or sieve. Freeze in an ice-cube tray.

It was at this stage that I started to add some fresh herbs to Helena's meals. During the summer I am constantly in and out of our garden picking over the herbs to add to our meals. So even if you don't grow your own, whenever you buy some fresh herbs for your own cooking (only fresh, not dried) why not start adding some to your child's meal? Make sure that the herbs are well washed and very finely chopped, and at first add only a very small amount (about ½ teaspoon per four ice-cubes for example). Helena loved potato, peas and mint as she did courgette, carrot, beans and mint. Other herby favourites included parsley, potato and carrot; cauliflower, broccoli, pepper, tomato and parsley; cauliflower, potato and chives; and carrot, broccoli, tomato and marjoram.

However, her all-time favourite was the most exotic and something I was very surprised that she liked. This only came about because I was making some marinated vegetables for a starter – and it just shows how much more open babies are to new tastes than we give them credit for!

Roasted red pepper, courgette and tomato with basil

1 red pepper
1 medium courgette
4–6 tomatoes
fresh basil

or
1 roasted pepper ice cube
2 courgette ice-cubes
2 tomato ice-cubes
fresh basil

Cut the pepper in half, deseed and core and cut into quarters. Place skin side up under a pre-heated grill and grill until skins start to blacken. Remove the skins and then chop the flesh. Purée with a little boiled water. Cook the courgette and tomato as in earlier recipes. Mix 1 dessertspoon of the roasted red pepper with 2 dessertspoons of courgette and an equal amount of tomato, add a teaspoonful of finely chopped basil and mix well. Add a little plain baby rice until you have a texture that your baby will like. Delicious!

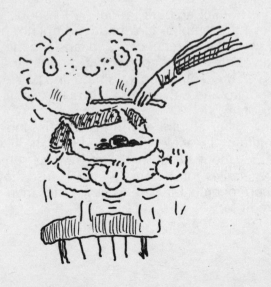

I'm afraid that when you taste baby food as good as this it really does make you wonder what on earth they do to the baby food that you get in most jars to make it taste so awful. I really would be most interested to actually go around a factory that produces baby food to find out how presumably perfectly normal ingredients manage to end up tasting so horrible. Nothing you ever make at home tastes that bad and even though most home-made baby food tastes bland to the average adult palate, it certainly still tastes of real food! However, when you start to be able to use herbs and get to the recipes like roasted red pepper, the main problem is making sure that it's the baby who gets fed and not the person feeding her!

By the way, I'm not suggesting that the last recipe is the sort that you can fit into your everyday busy routine. Obviously once the ice-cubes are in the freezer it is very easy to make up, but even easy recipes like this one that don't really take very long are just not practical to make on an everyday basis. Try it and neither you nor your baby will end up being happy. Babies always wake at the wrong moment so if yours should give you the luxury of a little rest period – rest! Only attempt this recipe when someone else is in charge of baby (then a little cooking can be quite restful).

Being the middle of summer we were also able to introduce Helena to a range of fresh fruits, but although I did prepare these a few times I felt that in essence the range of commercially made fruit purées that you can obtain is probably worth considering, especially if you were preparing these dishes in the winter months.

Apricot

Apricots mix well with other fruits so try your baby with apple and apricot and apricot and pear.

4 fresh apricots

Cut each apricot in half and remove the stone. If it does not come away, just leave it in and remove after cooking. (This applies to peaches as well.) Place in the top of a steamer and steam until soft (about 8–10 minutes). Cool and remove the skins (and stone if necessary). Purée.

Peach

Helena always liked peach and banana as well.

2 peaches

Cut each peach in half and remove the stone. Place in the top of a steamer and cook for 8–10 minutes until very soft. Remove the skin (and stone if necessary) and purée.

Melon

This is a very liquidy purée and I found that Helena much preferred it mixed with baby rice or as melon and banana.

half of a sweet ripe melon

Remove the seeds and scoop out the flesh. Place in a steamer and cook for 5 minutes. Purée.

Strawberry

Most of the advice to mothers is that berry fruit should not be given until the child is six months old. However, I did give Helena some strawberry purée when she was about five and a half months old. This was mainly because the strawberry season was fast drawing to a close and I did want to try her on them. But please be careful as the strawberry is one fruit that in some people does cause an allergic reaction.

200–250g (8–10 oz) strawberries

Hull the strawberries and slice if large, otherwise just cut in two. Place in the top of a steamer and cook for 3–5 minutes. Purée and put through a mouli or sieve.

Helena really loved these and had no reaction to them so we started to mix this purée with others – she loved anything with strawberry in it! Strawberry and apple with baby rice became a breakfast favourite; strawberry, melon and mint her favourite dessert. But then she wasn't averse to strawberry and banana for tea either!

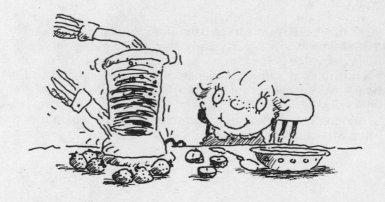

Fresh O.J. and rusk

Don't forget that freshly squeezed fruit juices are also a source of vitamins for your child. This is another breakfast favourite of Helena's. By the way, I was under the impression that small babies generally didn't like citrus fruits, the taste being too sour or sharp for them – James hadn't liked freshly squeezed orange juice as a baby. However, our friend Louise told me that she always gave her boys fresh orange juice every morning and they loved it! So when Helena came along we tried again, however this time we sieved it first (as advised by Louise) and yes, she loved it! James was also now a big fan, so our problem had not been that he didn't like the taste but that he didn't like the little bits in it. You live and learn.

> 1½ rusks (make sure it is a low-sugar, gluten-free variety)
> freshly squeezed orange juice – either from a carton or an orange!

Crumble the rusk and sieve the juice if necessary. Mix enough of the juice into the rusk to make a consistency that your baby will enjoy.

You can also use a crumbled rusk to mix with other fruit or vegetable purées instead of baby rice. Remember, however, that even the low-sugar variety has a sugar content while plain baby rice is sugar free – so better for your baby's teeth, even if there is still no evidence of them yet! Teeth can be harmed even before they appear, so take care of them for your baby.

Another recipe that I found was very popular which uses a juice was this next one.

Swede and apple baby rice

1 small swede

or
3–5 swede ice-cubes
freshly pressed apple juice
plain baby rice

Prepare the swede as in previous recipe (see page 37) or defrost the swede ice-cubes. Mix together with some apple juice and baby rice to produce a consistency that your baby will enjoy.

Travelling with baby

Whenever you take your baby out it always involves a lot of planning and preparation even for the smallest journey, so it is no wonder that many parents feel that they really don't want to take their new member of the family on holiday – the work involved seems to out-weigh the pleasures of the holiday. However, even at this tender age babies do enjoy the change in their routine and seem to take pleasure in the new scenery and people they meet when travelling, so I feel that even if it is not really a 'holiday' in the truest sense of the word for mum and dad, it is still a break and therefore will do everyone a little good. When James was four and a half months old and Andy was abroad on business, my mother and I took a lovely trip up north to see relations. We travelled slowly, stopping mainly at Travelodges when we were breaking a trip between relatives, and we all had a lovely time, taking in the Lake District, the Yorkshire Moors (to see where 'Heartbeat' is filmed), Whitby (to see Dracula's hiding place and where we had the best fish and chips I have ever had in my whole life) and York as well.

When Helena was a similar age we went as a family

on a little tour taking in Somerset, Dorset and Devon, again staying mainly at Travelodges and this time, to entertain James, visiting theme parks such as Crinkly Bottom, Monkeyworld, Paulton Park and beautiful Marwell Zoo. Lots of fun was had by all.

So on both trips, although they were still very reliant on their milk feeds, both children were also experimenting with different foods. Our friends Lucy and Chris took their son Christian on a canal boat when he was very young (and not crawling) so it is perfectly feasible to travel with baby. In fact Christian is one of the most well-travelled children I know, his experiences varying from camping to long-haul flights (Oman). I think they left him behind when visiting New York as I remember the postcard saying 'In the city that never sleeps – Lucy and Chris are!', and from our own experience when we get away from the children sleep is a very high priority.

When we are travelling we do try and keep to roughly the same routine that we have at home although we did change this a little in the evening so that our normal routine of 'Tea, Play, Bath, Books, Bed' became 'Tea, Play, Bath, Pub, Bed!' which was a change that everyone enjoyed (so much by James that he wanted to continue with it when we returned home).

If you are breastfeeding you are definitely at an advantage when travelling as you are always prepared for your baby's request to be fed. However, it becomes more difficult when you have to sterilise bottles and prepare milk feeds. You have two options: either take an appropriate sterilising kit with you or use disposable bottles (if you choose this route I suggest you practise using these at home first – we tried them but found that the bottles often leaked. However, other people I know have used them very successfully). For the actual journey take sterilised bottles and either milk powder and a flask of cooled, boiled water or cartons of pre-prepared milk feed. Don't keep warm, pre-prepared milk feeds in a flask as this could lead to food poisoning. Make sure that you have plenty of drinks available for your baby as travelling will make him thirsty.

Cans or jars of baby food are very useful, especially fruit, breakfast or yoghurt preparations as babies will happily eat these cold. I used to sterilise spoons and then wrap them in cling film or keep them in a container with a tight-fitting lid in sterilising solution and rinse with cooled, boiled water to use.

Bananas come in very useful when travelling as they are usually readily available at many cafés, service stations, etc. If you are not using the motorways to travel, supermarkets with cafés are an excellent choice as they often have a good choice of baby food and will warm it if necessary. For bigger babies who don't need food puréed, a portion of a parent's baked potato with cheese, mashed to baby's requirements, is a good choice, or simple sandwiches followed by a yoghurt or fruit.

3. Broadening the menu
   (six months to one year)

There is an enormous difference between the six-month-old baby and the one-year-old child. At six months old you will hopefully be able to put your youngster into a highchair at last – which in itself makes a lot of difference to mealtimes. But at one year old your child should not only be sitting in his highchair but will hopefully be feeding himself and eating the same meals as the rest of the family. Again individual children vary in the age at which they reach these achievements but what a difference it makes to their poor parents' lives when they do. For me one of the real highlights is being able to put away the sterilising unit – no more making up milk feeds or sterilising bottles. Bliss! I really look forward to the day when we can travel with the minimum of luggage again. No travelling cots, highchairs or pushchairs. What a difference it will make. Of course these could be left at home, but they can make all the difference between an enjoyable trip and a just plain exhausting one for the poor parents – for me, I really like not having to sleep with the baby and not having a wriggling infant sitting on my knee when trying to eat. Therefore I just get on with loading the car up. However, from one year old you could really manage with only a baby's cutlery and bib, and even these can be done without if really necessary.

At six months old when the baby is generally able to get around and will put everything he comes across in his mouth, there really is no point in continuing to sterilise his bowls and spoons. I also think that this is a good time to change over to a soft plastic bib, preferably with sleeves. It saves on the washing as these bibs can just be wiped down and left to dry. Babies vary a lot as to what age they will still allow you to feed them, but from quite an early age you will find the baby trying to grab the spoon off you. However, even just giving the baby a spoon and using one yourself won't really help you with some babies as they just throw whichever spoon they have on the floor and go for the one you have, and then after wrenching this from your hand (it's amazing how such a small creature can have such a grip) they throw that on the floor and battle recommences! The sooner you introduce your baby to finger food the better for your sanity. Then while he grapples with this you can try to get some of the real food down him. It can be a very difficult time. You want to get as much food into your sweetheart as possible, while baby is just intent on having a good time. It is generally a mucky experience which gets even worse when you bravely let your child have control of the bowl. Generally the food ends up all over the baby and the floor, but at least the child is enjoying his food! (Which is more than can be said for mother who is constantly worrying about whether the child is getting enough food to keep him alive. Don't panic!)

In a vain attempt to keep Helena's food in her bowl long enough for some to find its way to her mouth, it was at this stage I went out and bought one of those bowls that has a suction ring on it and therefore can be attached to the tray on the highchair – but these are no match for the average baby who will quickly pull it off! Luckily this stage only lasts a couple of weeks anyway. Eventually the baby does work out that the food is even more interesting if squeedged through the fingers and then stuffed in the mouth. Babies love trying to manipulate their environment – it is taken as a great challenge to chase every pea around the bowl until captured and painfully transferred to that waiting mouth – and the pleasure that babies have when they realise that they can actually transfer food from the bowl via this spoon (which so far has only been used for digging in the food and generally as a catapult) to their mouths has to be seen to be believed.

Now that the baby has reached the stage when they will accept some texture in their meals it is also the time to start to broaden their menus. At this age babies do vary and while some will still only accept very smooth purées others will be chewing at finger foods. If your child is still having very smooth purées try adding just a very small amount of grated food to the meal as well. Then gradually just add a little more grated or mashed food. (But don't push too hard, many babies much prefer smooth purées, so you do have to work very hard to get them to accept any lumps in their food – just take it slowly and they will eventually adjust.) Then you can start just to purée half of their meal while chopping up the remainder and then mixing it in. Keep reducing the amount that is puréed until your child will accept food that is just chopped or mashed. Still continue with their breastfeeds or one pint (20 fl oz or 500ml) of formula milk. If using formula it is time now to change to the 'follow-on' milk for your brand; this ensures that your child receives enough iron in her diet which is very important at this stage of growth. You can now start to use cow's milk in cereals and in cooking. Now is the time to introduce the yoghurts and fromage frais from the chilled cabinets. There are some, made from wholemilk, which are aimed specifically at babies. However, you can use normal yoghurts but don't go for the low-fat ones unless you have a very obese baby. You are still aiming to get a lot of calories into your child and especially if your child has a small appetite or is a very picky eater this is very important and these products can be very useful in this way. When Helena was going through the stage of fighting mother with every spoonful to go in her mouth, it was reassuring to know that in a few spoonfuls of fromage frais were virtually a hundred calories – the equivalent of a whole bottle of her milk. The only worrying factor about these yoghurts and fromage frais is the amount of sugar in most of them – even if flavoured only with fruit juices or purée the amount can still be quite high. Although the sugar in fruit is not considered as bad for you as refined sugar, when it is concentrated it becomes just as harmful to teeth, so do keep an eye on the amount you give your baby and keep them for meal-times. I did try both of my two on different natural yoghurts mixed with varying fruit purées but they thought this was yeuuch! – even Greek yoghurt which I adore on morning muesli. *C'est la vie*. However, at least once they are eating yoghurts it is something else which is easily available when travelling (a banana or part of a cheese sandwich followed by a yoghurt is acceptable to most babies and relatively easy to obtain) thus making life that little bit simpler.

Cheese plays a big part in our children's lives – both of mine have been very keen on grated cheese – and the sooner you get them on to little sandwiches the better. Many babies also love toast with just a little butter or soft margarine and a scraping of Marmite. You can now introduce different cereals to your baby – hot oat cereal and wheat biscuits seem to be the favourites with most mums (mainly because of the extra milk you can mix with them thereby increasing the nutrition of the meal). You can now introduce different meats and white fish to your baby too. Get them and their digestive system used to these and then introduce them to beans and pulses and oily fish.

By the age of one there is really very little that your child cannot eat, the main exceptions being foods that have a higher risk of carrying food poisoning, such as shellfish, partly cooked eggs and soft cheeses, and food which can cause your baby to choke, such as nuts.

Of course it is up to you to still ensure that your child is getting a balanced diet – fruit and vegetables still play a very important part. It is also important that you make a point of including iron-rich foods in your child's diet as many children do suffer from a lack of iron. And although energy foods are required to meet your child's growth requirements, these should not be in the form of lots of chips or sweets and biscuits. That is not to say that these foods have no place in their diets but for the sake of their health should be restricted.

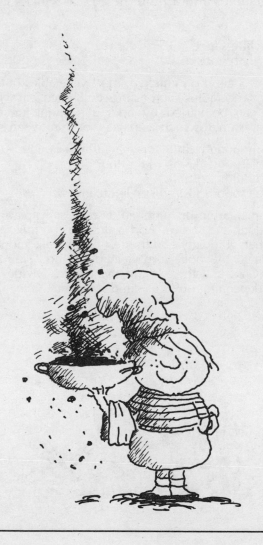

Sauces

It is useful to have a few sauces already made up and stored in the freezer. They can then be quickly defrosted and served either with fresh vegetables or with vegetables and a little meat or as sauces for pasta.

Creamy white sauce
Makes 4–6 portions

This sauce is good on chicken, most vegetables but particularly green vegetables such as broccoli, excellent with white fish and can be varied by adding a sprinkling of finely chopped fresh herbs such as parsley or mint when serving.

1 tablespoon (15ml) soft margarine or butter
1 tablespoon (15ml) plain flour
200ml (8 fl oz) milk
2 tablespoons (30ml) single cream

Melt the margarine or butter in a small saucepan and then add the flour and stir in. Add a little of the milk and keep stirring, then gradually add the rest of the milk and stir while you bring to the boil, turn heat down and simmer for 2 minutes. Cool and then stir in the cream. Divide into 4–6 portions depending on your child's appetite. Freeze.

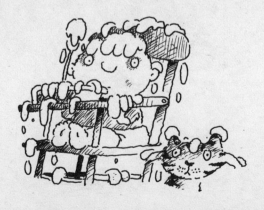

Cheesy sauce
Makes 4–6 portions

This sauce is good with fish or chicken, with many vegetables but is particularly good with pasta.

> 1 tablespoon (15ml) soft margarine or butter
> 1 tablespoon (15ml) plain flour
> 200ml (8 fl oz) milk
> 25g (1 oz) grated cheese such as cheddar or gruyère

Melt the margarine or butter in a small saucepan and stir in the flour, add a little of the milk and then while continuing to stir gradually add the rest of the milk. Bring to the boil and then turn the heat down and gently simmer for 2 minutes, add the cheese and stir until it has melted. Divide into 4–6 portions depending on your child's appetite and freeze what is not used.

Tomato and cheese sauce
Makes 2–3 portions

Excellent with pasta but also good on fish or pork dishes.

> 2 large tomatoes
> knob of butter or soft margarine
> 2 tablespoons (30ml) mascarpone or curd cheese
> 50g (2 oz) grated cheddar cheese

Firstly skin the tomatoes by covering with boiling water and leaving for 1–2 minutes, then cool and slip off the skins. Cut in half and take out the core and seeds. Chop the flesh up roughly. Melt the butter or margarine and gently fry the tomatoes for 2–3 minutes before adding the cheeses. Stir until cheeses melt. Put through a sieve or mouli to make a smooth sauce. Divide into 2–3 portions and freeze the unused sauce.

Baby tomato sauce
Makes 4–6 portions

Great with everything!

> 1 small onion, chopped
> 1 dessertspoon (10ml) olive or sunflower oil
> 400g can tomatoes
> pinch of dried oregano or chopped fresh marjoram

Fry the onion gently in the oil for 5 minutes or until soft but not colouring. Add the tomatoes (including the juice) and herbs. Simmer for 10 minutes and then put through a sieve or mouli. Divide into 4–6 portions and freeze whatever isn't used.

Vegetable sauce
Makes 6–8 portions

This sauce was developed because neither of my two little monkeys will eat mushrooms unless well disguised! It is very good with pasta, chicken, lamb or pork.

> 1 leek, cleaned, thinly sliced
> 1 courgette, ends removed and chopped
> 100–125g (4–5 oz) mushrooms, cleaned and sliced
> 1 carrot, chopped
> 25g (1 oz) butter or soft margarine
> 400g can tomatoes
> sprinkling finely chopped parsley (optional)

Cook the leek, courgette, mushrooms and carrot in the butter or margarine for 10 minutes until just starting to soften and colour. Add the tomatoes and simmer for 10 minutes. Cool and then stir in parsley if desired. Put through a sieve or mouli to get a smooth sauce. Divide into 6–8 portions and freeze for future use.

Chicken dishes

Chicken in green sauce
Makes 2–3 portions

    1 small chicken breast, boned and skinned, chopped
       into cubes
    few broccoli florets (about 75g or 3 oz)
    milk
    1 tablespoon (15ml) mascarpone or curd cheese

Put the chicken and broccoli into a small saucepan and just cover with milk. Bring to the boil and then just simmer until soft (about 10 minutes). When ready drain, reserving the milk. Purée. Put back in the pan with the cheese and 2 tablespoons of the saved milk. Stir while heating, then when the cheese has melted, remove from heat. Add more milk if you want to thin it down a little. Divide into 2–3 portions and freeze.

Chickenballs
Makes about 12 balls

Although I suppose you could make this recipe without a food processor (you could grate the chicken) I wouldn't bother! But if you do have one it is extremely quick and easy to make. You could also make chicken burgers by following the recipe and then flattening the balls into little burger shapes – you would need to turn them half way through cooking. In some supermarkets you can now get chicken mince so you could substitute this for the chicken breasts.

  2 chicken breasts (about 300g or 12 oz), boned and
    skinned
  2 spring onions, finely chopped
  3 tablespoons (45ml) fresh breadcrumbs
  1 small egg, beaten
  flour to coat
  oil for frying

Place the chicken in a food processor and process until finely chopped. Add the spring onions, breadcrumbs and egg and process briefly (the mixture should come together in a sticky ball). With your hands shape into about 12 little balls and coat with flour. Fry for 6–8 minutes until golden brown and cooked.

Cheesy chicken and peas
Makes 2 portions

  1 tablespoon (15ml) frozen peas
  1 small cooked chicken breast, boned and skinned
  2 portions cheesy sauce (see page 61)

Cook the peas either in a microwave or small saucepan. Either chop or shred the chicken (as preferred by your child). Drain the peas then return them to cooking dish with the chicken and sauce. Warm through thoroughly and serve.

Undercover chicken
Makes 1 portion

> 1 portion of cheesy chicken and peas
> 1 tablespoon (15ml) cornflakes, crushed

Pre-heat the oven to 180°C/350°F/Gas 4. In a small greased oven-proof dish place the portion of cheesy chicken and peas. Cover with the cornflakes and then bake for 20 minutes.

Chicken Veronique
Makes 2 portions

> 1 small cooked chicken breast, boned and skinned
> 2 portions creamy white sauce (see page 60)
> 6 muscat grapes, halved, seeded and skinned

Chop the chicken into small cubes or strips as preferred by your child, mix with the creamy white sauce and the grapes. Gently heat through in either a microwave or small saucepan and serve.

Sweet and sour chicken
Makes 2–4 portions

This recipe is an ideal introduction to more exotic tastes. Start by only using 1 tablespoon of soy sauce and then add more next time you make it. Helena, of course, has enjoyed this many times but the big breakthrough has just happened – at long last James has decided that he likes it too! (It's a miracle – put the flags out!) He decided that he would eat this with chopsticks and actually polished the lot off – mother was so excited that she had to ring daddy and tell him. With Helena breaking new ground and bringing the number of steps she had walked to seven, it was a bit of a record-breaking day.

1 small chicken breast, boned and skinned
1 tablespoon (15ml) cornflour
1 egg white, whisked
oil for frying
1 carrot, cut into matchsticks
2 tablespoons (30ml) sweetcorn
1 teaspoon (5ml) groundnut or sunflower oil

Sauce
1–2 tablespoons (15–30ml) soy sauce
1 tablespoon (15ml) orange or pineapple juice
1 tablespoon (15ml) tomato ketchup
3–4 tablespoons (45–60ml) water (depending on how much soy sauce you have used)
1 teaspoon (5ml) cornflour

Cut the chicken up into thin strips. Mix the tablespoon of cornflour with the beaten egg and coat each chicken strip with this. Fry until golden brown. Remove from the pan and drain. Now in another pan, stir fry the carrot in the teaspoon of groundnut or sunflower oil for 3 minutes and then add the sweetcorn. Mix together the sauce ingredients and add to the pan. Cook for 2 minutes and then add the cooked chicken, heat through and serve.

Chicken and tomato risotto
Makes 2–4 portions

> 2 tomatoes
> knob butter or soft margarine
> 1 small cooked chicken breast, boned and skinned
> 2 portions baby tomato sauce (see page 62)
> 2–3 tablespoons (30–45ml) cooked long grain rice

Skin the tomatoes by covering with boiling water and leaving for 1–2 minutes. Peel off the skin and remove the core and seeds. Chop the flesh. Cook gently in the butter or margarine for 2–3 minutes until soft. Chop the chicken and mix all ingredients together. Gently heat through in a microwave or small saucepan.

Pork

One of the good things that has come out of the BSE scare is many more varieties of meat are regularly available minced. Any of these recipes that use either minced pork or lamb could have beef mince substituted instead.

Pork Italienne
Makes 2–4 portions

> 100g (4 oz) pork mince
> 1 carrot, finely chopped
> 4 portions baby tomato sauce (see page 62)
> 50g (2 oz) Organix baby pasta shapes

Put the pork in a small frying pan and gently fry – you want to release any fat from the meat so that you can pour it off. When drained, add the carrot and mix in the tomato sauce, cover and cook gently for 15 minutes, cool and purée briefly. Meanwhile cook the pasta shapes in boiling water for 10 minutes. Drain and mix with the meat sauce. Heat through thoroughly and serve.

Saucy pork
Makes 2–4 portions

> 100g (4 oz) pork mince
> 1 carrot, finely chopped
> 3 portions tomato and cheese sauce (see page 61)

Put the pork into a small frying pan and just cook gently to release any fat, then drain. Add the carrot and 6 tablespoons (90ml) water and then cover and simmer gently for 15 minutes. Drain and mix with the tomato and cheese sauce, purée briefly. Heat through thoroughly. Serve over rice or pasta.

Pork and leeks with pasta
Makes 2–4 portions

> 100g (4 oz) pork mince
> 1 small leek, cleaned and sliced thinly
> 4 portions vegetable sauce (see page 62)
> 50g (2 oz) Organix baby pasta shapes

Place the pork mince in a small frying pan and gently cook to release any fat, and drain. Add the leek and then mix in the vegetable sauce. Cover and then gently simmer for 15 minutes. Cool, purée briefly. Meanwhile cook the pasta shapes in boiling water for 10 minutes. Drain and mix with the pork and vegetable sauce. Heat thoroughly and serve.

Pork and beans
Makes 2–4 portions

> 100g (4 oz) pork mince
> 1 carrot, finely chopped
> 150g can baked beans in reduced-sugar sauce

Place the pork mince in a small frying pan and cook gently to release any fat, and drain. Add the carrot and 6 tablespoons (90ml) of water. Cover and then gently simmer for 15 minutes. Drain and purée briefly. Mix with the beans in their sauce (depending on your baby's preference you can mash these a little before adding), heat through thoroughly and serve.

Lamb

Although lamb is quite a fatty meat it also has a sweet flavour which is generally liked by children. Therefore, although not a dish you should serve every day, definitely one which should find a place in your menus.

In the late winter months we can see the sheep in the fields outside our home and soon I know we will have our first lambs of the season. James will be three this year and I know that at some point in the near future he is going to make the connection between the lamb he is eating and those animals in the fields. I really have no idea how he is going to react – it's something that I have not made a point of explaining. I don't have a problem with eating meat – only with the way that some livestock is treated during its life. However, many children are vegetarian in this modern day. I would prefer it if my children do eat meat – it is a very good source of iron which, nowadays, many children are deficient in. There are also many lovely meat dishes which I enjoy both cooking and eating, and as we like to eat as a family it will restrict my cooking if I can only cook vegetarian meals. But I can see that when a small child makes this connection between the meat they eat and the animals they see in the field it might well lead to that child becoming a vegetarian. Strangely for some people this realisation comes quite late in their childhood but it is at this point that the decision to turn vegetarian does occur.

Our friend Claire has been bringing Brendan up on a vegetarian diet – he was extremely surprised to be told that people eat meat from animals. After she had discussed this with him she then heard him running around saying 'You eat camel, you eat camel!' Being a logical child he had of course taken the next step and assumed that if people eat lamb or pork, why not camel? Why indeed? I don't know what we will be introducing our children to next, ostrich is already on our shelves. Why are we squeamish about eating some animals and not others?

Minty lamb with broccoli
Makes 2–4 portions

> 100g (4 oz) lamb mince
> 75g (3 oz) broccoli florets
> 3 portions creamy white sauce (see page 60)
> sprinkling finely chopped mint

Place the lamb mince in a small frying pan and cook gently to release any fat, and drain. Add 6 tablespoons (90ml) of water, cover and simmer gently for 5 minutes. Add the broccoli and continue simmering for another 10 minutes. Drain and purée briefly. Mix with the creamy white sauce and mint and heat through thoroughly. Serve with rice or potatoes.

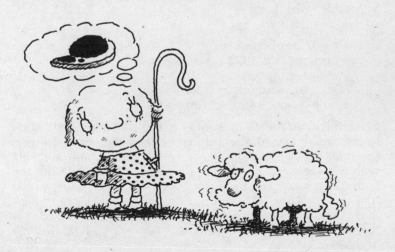

Scarborough lamb
Makes 2–4 portions

This recipe is a lovely mixture of lamb and herbs mixed with carrot and potato. Although I have used some dried herbs here, if you are the proud possessor of a herb garden you could use a mixture of herbs, such as parsley, sage, rosemary and thyme.

> 100g (4 oz) lamb mince
> 1 teaspoon (5ml) mixed herbs
> 1 carrot, finely chopped
> 150g (6 oz) potato, skinned and chopped

Place the lamb mince in a medium saucepan and gently cook to release any fat, and drain. Then add the herbs, carrot and potato to the saucepan and just cover with water. Bring to the boil, cover and simmer for 15–20 minutes until the potato is cooked through. Drain, reserving 1–2 tablespoons (15–30ml) of the cooking stock. Place this reserved stock with the meat and veg in a blender and purée briefly, serve.

Vegetables with lamb
Makes 2–4 portions

> 100g (4 oz) lamb mince
> 3 portions vegetable sauce (see page 62)
> 1 carrot, chopped
> 50g (2 oz) cauliflower florets
> 1 tablespoon (15ml) frozen peas

Place the lamb mince in a small frying pan and gently cook to release any fat, drain and just cover with water. Bring to the boil, cover and simmer for 15 minutes. Drain and mix with the vegetable sauce. Briefly purée. Meanwhile put the carrot in a saucepan and just cover with water, bring to the boil and cook for 10 minutes. Add the cauliflower and peas and cook for a further 5 minutes. Drain. Mix all ingredients together (mashing the vegetables if necessary), heat through and serve.

72

Fish

Try your children on white fish to start with. I found that my two were both very keen on lemon sole – but even though I was buying it in very small quantities it is still a more expensive option than cod, plaice or haddock, which are more readily available. After you have got your baby used to the taste of white fish then try her on an oily fish such as salmon or sardines. But of course whatever fish you are giving your baby it must be completely free of any bones. I think it is for this reason that many mothers are frightened to cook fish for their children. However, there are many cuts that are virtually boneless and very easy to cook. Of course your child might just not like the taste, for instance James will eat very little fish, while as long as the texture is right for her Helena will eat virtually any type! You can but try.

Cod in parsley sauce
Makes 2–3 portions

> 100g (4 oz) cod fillet, skinned
> 2 portions creamy white sauce (see page 60)
> sprinkling finely chopped parsley

Either cook the fish in your microwave oven according to the manufacturer's directions (which will take only a few minutes) or place on some oiled greaseproof paper and cook in the top of a steamer for 8–10 minutes (this depends on the thickness of your fillet). Flake the fish, making sure there are no bones present. Meanwhile heat the sauce either in the microwave or in a small saucepan, add the parsley and pour over the fish.

Cod in cheese and tomato sauce
Makes 2–3 portions

> 100g (4 oz) cod fillet, skinned
> 2 portions tomato and cheese sauce (see page 61)

Either cook the fish in a microwave according to the manufacturer's instructions (which will only take a few minutes) or
place on some buttered greaseproof paper and cook in the
top of a steamer for 7–10 minutes (this will depend on the
thickness of your fish fillet). Flake the fish, checking that no
bones are present. Heat the sauce in a microwave or in a
small saucepan and serve mixed in with the fish.

Plaice with peas in cheese sauce
Makes 2–3 portions

> 100g (4 oz) plaice fillet, skinned
> 1 tablespoon (15ml) frozen peas
> 2 portions cheesy sauce (see page 61)

Cook the plaice fillet either in your microwave oven according to the manufacturer's directions or place on some oiled
greaseproof paper and cook in the top of a steamer for 8–10
minutes. Flake the fish. Meanwhile heat the peas and cheese
sauce (either using the microwave or in a small saucepan).
Mix all the ingredients together and serve.

Lemon sole
Makes 1–2 portions

Both of my two monkeys love lemon sole cooked like this but I do occasionally serve it with creamy white sauce (using two portions) and skinned halved grapes – this is my version of lemon sole Veronique.

    100g (4 oz) lemon sole fillet
    squeeze lemon juice

Cook the lemon sole using a microwave (which will take 3–4 minutes) or by placing it on a sheet of buttered greaseproof paper and cooking in the top of a steamer for 8–10 minutes. Remove the skin and flake the fish. Add just a tiny squeeze of lemon juice before serving.

Beans and lentils

From the age of about eight months you can start to add pulses to your child's menus. The reason for starting a little later with pulses is that they are very fibrous and a very young child's digestive system is too immature to cope with them. Also as they are so fibrous a child can only eat them in small quantities and will not get the required amount of calories from small quantities.

Butter beans in cheese sauce
Makes 2–4 portions

> 150g can butter beans
> 2 portions of cheesy sauce, heated through and then cooled (see page 61)

Drain the butter beans and wash with running water. According to your child's likes either serve whole or mashed into the sauce, or if necessary you can purée with the sauce.

Butter bean salad
Makes 2–4 portions

> 150g can butter beans
> 2 tablespoons (30ml) natural fromage frais
> sprinkling fresh finely chopped parsley, chives or mint

Drain the butter beans and wash under running water. Mix with the fromage frais and sprinkle with herbs. Purée briefly or mash if necessary for your child.

Lentil and potato mash
Makes 2–4 portions

> 25g (1 oz) red lentils
> 200g (8 oz) potato, peeled and cut into cubes
> 375ml (15 fl oz) water or home-made stock

Put all the ingredients into a medium saucepan, bring to the boil and then cover and simmer gently, stirring occasionally for about 20 minutes. Drain, then purée or lightly mash together. (By the age of one you can actually leave the potato unmashed if your baby can handle the size of potato cubes.) As baby gets older you can jazz this up by adding a little Marmite or tomato ketchup and serving with some cheese.

Cheese and tomato lentils
Makes 2–4 portions

> 25g (1 oz) red lentils
> 2 tomatoes
> 25g (1 oz) grated cheddar cheese
> sprinkling fresh finely chopped parsley (optional)

Place the lentils in a small saucepan and cover with water, bring to the boil and then simmer for 15–20 minutes until cooked – stir occasionally and add more water if necessary. Meanwhile cover the tomatoes with boiling water, leave for two minutes and then slip off the skins. Halve, remove the core and seeds, and chop up the flesh. When the lentils are cooked, cool and then mix with the tomatoes, cheese and parsley.

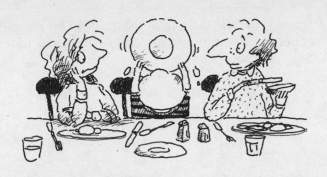

4. Meals with the family

In our busy lives it can sometimes be difficult for everyone to sit down and eat their meals together. Since, however, it is my belief that this is one of the cornerstones of the family I do make a point of making sure that whenever possible we do eat all together. In our household as long as daddy is not away on business we always have proper Saturday and Sunday lunches, where the table is set and the food is put out on serving dishes, and it is obvious that both James and Helena enjoy these occasions. Of course it does restrict what you can put on the menu when you have fussy children to cater for too – but mum and dad keep Friday night free for dishes that the children won't eat, for example curry.

I do think that life is too short to cook more than one dish at lunchtime so I always opt for a meal that can be eaten by the whole family. If your baby is under six months old just purée some of the vegetables you are cooking to accompany the main meal for her, but if over this age she can have a little of everything. The main points to watch are not to add any extra salt to meals for baby and to cut up or purée the food to a texture acceptable to your child. Mum and dad will have to add their seasoning at the table. The recipes in this section will feed two adults and either two toddlers or a baby and toddler.

Asparagus risotto

Risottos are popular in our house and here are two of our favourites – the asparagus risotto was the first proper meal that Helena ever had.

    large knob of butter
    150g (6 oz) risotto rice (arborio or carnerolli)
    600ml (1¼ pints) chicken or vegetable stock
    250g (10 oz) asparagus tips
    50g (2 oz) grated cheese – preferably parmesan but
        cheddar or gruyère work well

In a medium saucepan melt the butter and stir in the rice, making sure it is well coated with the melted butter. Add one third of the stock (200ml or 8 fl oz) and simmer until the stock is absorbed. Then add half of the remaining stock and again cook until the rice has absorbed the liquid. Add the remaining stock and cook until the stock has been virtually absorbed and the rice is cooked (this should take in total about 15–18 minutes). Meanwhile either microwave or steam the asparagus tips until tender, this should take about 4–8 minutes depending on the thickness of the spears. Finally stir into the rice the asparagus and the cheese and serve.

Baked ham and pea risotto

Don't worry about the sherry in this recipe as the alcohol is evaporated off and just leaves the lovely flavouring. However, if you prefer not to add it just increase the amount of stock by 100ml (4 fl oz)

  50g (2 oz) butter
  1 onion, chopped
  150g (6 oz) risotto rice (arborio or carnerolli)
  100g (4 oz) frozen peas
  500ml (1 pint) chicken or ham stock
  100ml (4 fl oz) medium-dry sherry
  50g (2 oz) grated cheddar cheese
  150g (6 oz) wafer-thin honey roast ham, shredded

Pre-heat the oven to 150°C/300°F/Gas 2. Melt the butter in a shallow oven-proof pan and gently fry the onion, until it softens and is just starting to colour. Add the rice and stir, making sure it is well coated with the butter. Add the peas, stock and sherry and bring to the boil, then immediately transfer, uncovered, to the oven. Cook for 30 minutes, add the cheese and ham, stir through and cook for a further 5 minutes. Serve.

Pork Creole

3 boneless pork shoulder steaks
1 onion, chopped
1 red pepper, chopped
1 carrot, chopped
1 tablespoon (15ml) olive oil
2 sticks celery, thinly sliced
400g can chopped tomatoes
sprinkling mild jalapeño pepper sauce (for adults)

Pre-heat the oven to 180°C/350°F/Gas 4. Place the pork steaks in a shallow casserole dish. Cook the onion, pepper and carrot in the oil until they start to colour, mix with the celery and tomatoes and spoon over the steaks. Cover and cook in the oven for 1¼–1½ hours until pork is tender. Divide one steak between the children and add some of the vegetables. Divide the remaining steaks and vegetables between the adults and sprinkle liberally with the jalapeño sauce.

Stuffed chicken breasts

3 chicken breasts, boned and skinned
50g (2 oz) gruyère cheese, grated
50g (2 oz) wafer-thin honey roast ham, shredded
100ml (4 fl oz) dry vermouth or chicken stock
sprinkling fresh finely chopped parsley or chives

Pre-heat the oven to 180°C/350°F/Gas 4. Make a lengthways slit along each chicken breast and stuff with the cheese and ham, secure with cocktail sticks and put in a small oven-proof dish. Pour in the vermouth or stock and cover tightly. Cook in the pre-heated oven for 45 minutes–1 hour until chicken is cooked. Remove the cocktail sticks. Divide one chicken breast between the children and sprinkle with parsley or chives. Divide the remaining chicken between the adults.

Braised lamb with beans

This is a lovely recipe for lamb that I have adapted from an old French recipe. It is one of our children's favourites. It is important to start this recipe the day before you want to serve it.

200g (8 oz) flageolet beans
600g (1¼ lb) braising or casserole lamb, cubed
2 tablespoons (30ml) olive oil
2 onions, sliced
2 cloves garlic, crushed
1 tablespoon (15ml) plain flour
500ml (1 pint) lamb stock
3 sprigs rosemary
2 bay leaves
1 tablespoon (15ml) fresh finely chopped thyme
400g can chopped tomatoes

Bring the beans to the boil in a large saucepan of water. Boil for 10 minutes then turn off and leave to soak overnight in the cooking water.

Pre-heat the oven to 150°C/300°F/Gas 2. Quickly fry the lamb in the oil until starting to colour and then transfer to a hob-proof casserole dish. Fry the onion and garlic in the same pan you used to fry the lamb. When starting to colour add to the casserole. Stir in the flour and add the stock, drained beans and herbs. Place on the hob and bring to the boil. Cover and transfer to the pre-heated oven. Cook for 1½ hours before adding tomatoes (and the juice from the can) and cooking for a further hour.

Granny's chicken casserole

3 chicken breasts, boned and skinned
large knob of butter
1 tablespoon (15ml) olive oil
1 onion, chopped
2 cloves garlic, crushed
1 tablespoon (15ml) plain flour
375ml (15 fl oz) chicken stock
3 tablespoons (45ml) tomato purée
sprinkling of mixed herbs
2 tablespoons (30ml) double cream or crème fraîche

Pre-heat the oven to 180°C/350°F/Gas 4. Fry the chicken breasts in the butter and oil until starting to brown. Transfer to a casserole dish. Fry the onion and garlic until starting to colour and also transfer to the casserole dish. Stir the flour into the frying pan and mix well with meat and onion juices. Add the stock, tomato purée and herbs to the cooking pan and bring to the boil. Pour over the chicken, cover and cook in the pre-heated oven for 1½ hours. Just before serving stir in the double cream or crème fraîche.

Normandy pheasant

This recipe is lovely to brighten up the winter months – it was the first proper meal that we ever gave to James and it is still a strong favourite. It can, of course, also be cooked substituting chicken or guinea fowl for the pheasant. The amount cooked here always leaves us with enough to make a soup as well – simply ensure that no bones are present and shred the meat, then purée the remains and make up to 500ml (1 pint) with chicken or vegetable stock. Purée again, heat through thoroughly and serve, giving you a lovely pheasant soup.

1 oven-ready pheasant
large knob of butter
65g (2½ oz) pancetta, cubed
1 onion, chopped
2 cloves garlic, crushed
200g (8 oz) cooking apples, cored, peeled and sliced
150ml (6 fl oz) dry cider
1 tablespoon (15ml) redcurrant jelly (optional)
125ml (5 fl oz) double cream
sprinkling fresh finely chopped parsley

Pre-heat the oven to 180°C/350°F/Gas 4. Fry the pheasant in the butter to just colour it. Transfer to a casserole dish. Then in the same frying pan cook the pancetta, onion and garlic, transfer to the casserole dish. Lastly quickly fry the apple in the pan (add a little more butter if necessary to stop the slices sticking). Add the cider and redcurrant jelly if using. Bring to the boil and then pour over the pheasant. Cover and cook for 1½ hours. Remove the pheasant and liquidise the sauce, mixing in the cream. Take as much meat off the pheasant as you can and mix into the sauce, gently reheat the meat and sauce. Sprinkle with parsley before serving.

Fish steaks

Do try and get your children to eat fish as it is a low-fat food that is full of vitamins. Don't just stop at the usual kinds such as cod or plaice but try them on some of the more exotic varieties such as tuna or swordfish; these fish are more expensive but well worth making into a special treat.

> 2 tablespoons (30ml) olive oil
> juice of 1 lemon
> sprinkling fresh parsley, thyme or marjoram
> 3 firm fish steaks, for example monkfish, tuna or
>   swordfish
> large knob of butter
> sprinkling mild jalapeño sauce (optional, for adults)

Mix the olive oil, lemon juice and herbs together and use to marinade the fish steaks. Leave for 1–2 hours, turning once if possible. Fry in the butter for 8–10 minutes until the fish is cooked. Add the marinade mixture and simmer for 1 minute. Remove any bones and flake one fish steak for the children, serve with marinade juices poured over. Divide the remaining fish and pan juices between the adults, sprinkling with the jalapeño sauce if using.

Salmon with watercress sauce

> 3 salmon steaks
> large knob of butter
> small bunch of watercress, washed
> 3 tablespoons (45ml) of fresh chopped parsley
> 125ml (5 fl oz) crème fraîche

Fry the salmon steaks gently in the butter for 12–15 minutes, turning once. Purée the watercress, parsley and crème fraîche and then heat gently in a small saucepan. Remove all bones from one of the salmon steaks and flake the fish, mix with 2 tablespoons of the sauce and serve to the children. Divide the remaining fish and sauce between the adults.

Fishycakes

400g (1 lb) potatoes, cooked and mashed with a knob
    of butter and 2 tablespoons (30ml) milk
400g (1 lb) fish, cooked and flaked
1 tablespoon (15ml) fresh finely chopped parsley
1 egg
4 slices bread, crumbed
a little oil for frying

Using your hands mix together the potato mash, fish and
parsley. Divide into 8 portions. Gently shape each portion
into little cakes. Break the egg into a saucer and beat gently.
Coat the fishycakes with egg and then breadcrumbs and fry
gently for about 4–5 minutes on each side. Fry them gently,
as you want them to be golden brown.

Fish crumble

   400g (1 lb) cod or salmon fillet
   juice of 1 lemon
   125ml (5 fl oz) fish stock
   2 leeks, finely sliced
   knob of butter
   1 tablespoon (15ml) plain flour
   150ml (6 fl oz) milk
   1 tablespoon (15ml) fresh finely chopped parsley
   3 slices bread, crumbed
   50g (2 oz) cheddar or gruyère cheese

Pre-heat the oven to 200°C/400°F/Gas 6. Place the fish fillets in a sauté pan which has a lid, pour in the lemon juice and fish stock, cover and poach gently for 10–12 minutes until the fish is cooked. Remove from the heat and if necessary remove any skin (flake the fish, checking for bones). Put the fish into a shallow casserole or gratin dish and save the stock. Gently fry the leek in the butter until starting to colour, then stir in the flour, and gradually blend in the milk. Add the stock that you cooked the fish in, and the parsley and mix well. Cook for a few minutes as the sauce thickens. Remove from the heat and stir into the fish. Sprinkle with the breadcrumbs and cheese and cook in the pre-heated oven for 20–25 minutes.

Lamb hot pot

400g (1 lb) potatoes, thinly sliced
1 onion, sliced
3–4 lamb loin or butterfly chops
3 lambs' kidneys (optional)
2 carrots, diced
200ml (8 fl oz) lamb stock
dash of Worcestershire sauce
1 teaspoon (5ml) tomato purée or ketchup
sprinkling of thyme
knob of butter, melted

Pre-heat the oven to 170°C/325°F/Gas 3. Put a layer of potatoes (leaving some for the top) and onion into a casserole dish, add the chops (and kidneys if using), add the carrots and then cover with the rest of the potato slices. Mix together the lamb stock, Worcestershire sauce, tomato purée or sauce and thyme. Pour into the casserole dish. Cover the top of the potato slices with the melted butter. Cover the casserole and cook in the pre-heated oven for 2 hours. Remove the cover and turn up the heat to 220°C/425°F/Gas 7 and cook for a further 15 minutes to brown the potatoes. When serving remove the meat from the bones before dishing up the children's portions to ensure that they do not get any bones.

Lamb noisettes

In the springtime nothing beats the taste of the new season's lamb; it is exceptionally sweet and tender. Again it was one of the first dishes that Helena had and proved to be very popular indeed. In this recipe I have used noisettes but you could equally use loin chops.

>   6 lamb noisettes
>   melted butter
>   sprinkling of fresh finely chopped mint

Place the lamb noisettes on a grill pan and brush with melted butter, sprinkle with mint and cook under a medium grill for about 6–8 minutes. Turn the noisettes over and again brush with melted butter and sprinkle with mint. Grill again for a further 5–7 minutes. Chop or cut up one noisette each for the children, dividing the other noisettes between the adults.

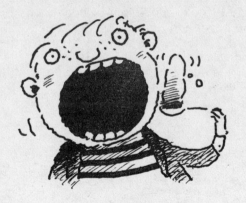

Egg and tomato scramble

Although neither of my two will currently eat eggs I am told that this recipe is very popular with children who do like eggs.

1 onion, chopped
1 tablespoon (15ml) olive oil
3–4 large ripe tomatoes (skinned if cooking for a baby)
6 eggs
knob of butter
1 clove garlic, crushed (optional)
squeeze of lemon juice

Fry the onion in the olive oil for a few minutes until soft and just starting to colour. Halve the tomatoes and take out the core and seeds. Thinly slice the tomatoes and put to one side. Beat the eggs and then melt the butter in the pan you have cooked the onions in. Add the tomatoes, egg and garlic (if using) to the onions and butter. Keep stirring the eggs to scramble them, cooking them until they are creamy and just starting to harden, then stir in the lemon juice and serve with toast triangles made from brown bread (or baby rice if cooking for a baby who doesn't eat toast yet).

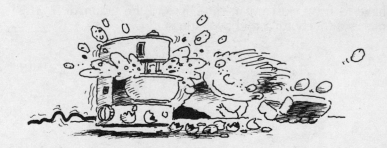

Baked avocado and chicken

3 chicken breast fillets, skinned and boned
1 tablespoon (15ml) olive oil
1 onion, chopped
2 celery sticks, thinly sliced
1 tablespoon (15ml) plain flour
250ml (½ pint) milk
1 large ripe avocado
juice of 1 lemon
3 slices bread, crumbed
50g (2 oz) cheddar or gruyère cheese, grated

Pre-heat the oven to 200°C/400°F/Gas 6. Firstly slice the chicken into strips and then fry in the oil until starting to colour, then remove to a shallow casserole dish or gratin dish. Add the onion and celery to the pan and cook until softened and just starting to colour, stir in the flour and gradually blend in the milk. Cook for 2 minutes while stirring, until sauce thickens. Halve the avocado, remove the stone and the skin, dice or thinly slice the flesh, mix in with the chicken and then add the sauce and lemon juice. Sprinkle with the breadcrumbs and cheese and cook in the pre-heated oven for 20–25 minutes until browning.

I often substitute a can of tuna (175g–200g) for the chicken in this recipe. This saves time if I'm in a hurry as you don't have to fry it, just put it directly into the gratin dish. This makes a lovely tuna and avocado gratin.

Ratatouille cheese crumble

If you are lucky enough to have children with fairly adventurous taste buds they will love this next recipe. In our household this recipe is loved by everyone – except James. You can, of course, just serve the ratatouille as a meal in itself and we have often had it with baked potatoes and grated cheese, or sometimes served on a bed of rice.

1 onion, chopped
1 clove garlic, crushed
1 red pepper, chopped
2 tablespoons (30ml) olive oil
1 courgette, cut into small chunks
1 aubergine, diced
400g can chopped tomatoes with basil
2 tablespoons (30ml) plain flour
4 tablespoons (60ml) oats
50g (2 oz) butter
50g (2 oz) grated cheddar or gruyère cheese

Pre-heat the oven to 200°C/400°F/Gas 6. Fry the onion, garlic and pepper in the oil for a few minutes until softening and just starting to colour, then add the courgette and aubergine and 1 tablespoon of water. Cover and cook gently for 10 minutes. Add the can of tomatoes and mix well. Place in a casserole dish and cover. Cook in the pre-heated oven for 30 minutes. Meanwhile prepare the crumble topping. Gently rub together the flour, oats and butter until they look like breadcrumbs. Stir in the cheese. After the ratatouille mixture has cooked for 30 minutes, uncover and top with the cheese crumble mixture, then cook uncovered for another 20–25 minutes until the crumble has browned.

Baked savoury cheese sandwich

Baked savoury sandwiches are usually well received by young children as the texture suits them, they are so easy to digest, and they also contain a lot of protein from the milk and eggs so it is a good meal for young children. Served with some broccoli or spinach (if your children eat spinach – I have not found many children who do like it) it makes a very good nutritious meal that is also very cheap to make.

Unfortunately although meals based on eggs are very nutritious, because of their cholesterol level, eggs should play a limited part in our children's diets – they are certainly not suitable for everyday consumption as was thought in the past. (I certainly remember the 'go to work on an egg' advertising campaign.)

> 5 slices bread, buttered
> 100g (4 oz) cheddar cheese, grated
> Marmite
> 300ml (12 fl oz) milk
> 2 eggs, beaten

Pre-heat the oven to 180°C/350°F/Gas 4. Cut each bread slice in half diagonally. Divide the cheese between half of the bread slices and spread the other halves with Marmite. Sandwich the bread slices together and cut each half in half again. (You'll now have 10 triangles.) Place in a buttered oven-proof gratin dish. Beat together the milk and eggs and pour over the sandwiches. Push the bread into the milk and egg mixture to ensure it gets well coated. Cook in the pre-heated oven for 30–40 minutes until risen and brown.

Tasty steak salad

When your children are into finger food we have found this recipe to be very popular as both the meat and vegetables are easily picked up with their fingers. I usually serve this with rice and peas. If your toddlers won't eat red pepper then you can omit it when cooking and just stir in some halved cherry tomatoes when serving. James likes tomato sauce mixed into his serving as well!

    200g (8 oz) rump steak, all excess fat removed
    1 tablespoon (15ml) soy sauce
    squeeze of lemon juice
    2 tablespoons (30ml) white wine, sherry or orange
      juice
    1 tablespoon (15ml) oil
    100g (4 oz) button mushrooms, halved
    1 red pepper, cored and seeded, then cut into strips
    1 little gem lettuce, stalk removed and leaves
      separated

Cut the steak into thin strips and put in a bowl with the soy sauce, lemon juice, white wine, sherry or orange juice and the oil. Cover and marinade for at least 2 hours or even overnight. Start to cook the meat 10 minutes before you wish to serve the salad. Pre-heat a large frying pan and then add the meat and marinade to the pan along with the mushrooms and red pepper. Stir fry for 2 minutes. Add 1 tablespoon water, cover and cook for a further 5 minutes. Uncover and stir in the lettuce leaves. Serve immediately.

Chicken in lemon yoghurt sauce

2 carrots, sliced
1 leek, halved lengthwise, cleaned and cut into thin strips
2 celery sticks, thinly sliced
1 tablespoon (15ml) oil or soft margarine
3 chicken breasts, skinned and boned
200ml (8 fl oz) chicken stock
juice of 1 lemon
3 tablespoons (45ml) natural Greek yoghurt

Place the carrots, leek and celery with the oil or margarine in a sauté pan which has a lid. Cook until starting to soften and just starting to colour. Place the chicken breasts on the vegetables. Mix together the chicken stock and the lemon juice and pour over the chicken breasts. Cover and cook for 15–20 minutes until the chicken is cooked through. Stir in the Greek yoghurt and heat through before serving.

Chicken in banana cream sauce

1 onion, finely chopped
1 tablespoon (15ml) oil
3 chicken breasts, skinned and boned
200ml (8 fl oz) chicken stock
2 bananas
3 tablespoons (45ml) crème fraîche

In a sauté pan which has a lid, fry the onion in the oil until just starting to colour, then add the chicken breasts and the chicken stock. Cover and gently cook for 15–20 minutes until the chicken is cooked through. Remove the chicken breasts and then liquidise the onion, cooking juices, bananas and crème fraîche. Return the liquidised sauce and the chicken to the pan and heat through before serving.

Cheese sauce

This recipe is for a cheese sauce which you can make thicker by adding the smaller amount of milk, or for a thinner sauce add the larger amount of milk. There is a large amount of cheese in this sauce, so it is very suitable for serving as a complete meal with some cooked vegetables and either a baked potato, some pasta or rice. However, I shall use it to make that classic childhood dish – a macaroni cheese.

50g (2 oz) butter or margarine
50g (2 oz) plain flour
400–500ml (16–20 fl oz) milk
100g (4 oz) grated cheddar cheese

Melt the butter or margarine in a small saucepan and then remove from the heat. Add the flour, stir well and return to the heat. Gradually blend in the milk, stirring continuously. When you have added all the milk continue to cook for a couple of minutes and then stir in the grated cheese. Continue to cook until the cheese has melted.

Macaroni cheese

There are many variations on this classic dish. I have often made it adding some cooked broccoli and cauliflower to the macaroni sauce, or alternatively adding some skinned, chopped tomatoes (or even a small can of chopped tomatoes) to the macaroni cheese mixture before baking.

200g (8 oz) quick cook macaroni
400ml (16 fl oz) cheese sauce (as above)
1 teaspoon (5ml) French mustard
knob of butter (for greasing)
3 slices of bread, crumbed
75g (3 oz) grated cheddar cheese

Pre-heat the oven to 180°C/350°F/Gas 4. Cook the macaroni in boiling water until just tender – about 4 minutes. Mix the cheese sauce with the French mustard and then the macaroni. Pour into a greased gratin dish and cover with the breadcrumbs and the cheese. Cook in the pre-heated oven for 30 minutes until the topping has browned.

Farmhouse pork stew

Start this recipe the day before you wish to serve it. Soak the beans overnight in a large bowl of cold water. Drain, rinse and then cook for 10 minutes in boiling water before draining and using.

    65g chopped pancetta (or chopped streaky bacon)
    1 onion, chopped
    2 sticks celery
    1 carrot, sliced
    1 tablespoon (15ml) oil
    400g (1 lb) pork casseroles cubes
    400g can chopped tomatoes
    100g (4 oz) dried butter beans
    sprinkling dried thyme

Pre-heat the oven to 170°C/325°F/Gas 3. Fry the pancetta, onion, celery and carrot in the oil for a few minutes to soften. Add the casserole meat and fry for a further 5 minutes until browned. Place in a casserole dish and add the tomatoes and butter beans. Sprinkle with thyme, then add enough boiling water to ensure that the beans are covered. Cover and cook in the pre-heated oven for 2 hours.

Beef olives

3 thin slices of topside of beef – you will probably have to ask your butcher for these
75g (3 oz) pork sausagemeat
1 small leek, halved lengthwise, cleaned and sliced thinly
1 tablespoon (15ml) sherry
glass of red wine (125ml)
125ml (5 fl oz) beef stock
1 tablespoon (15ml) tomato purée

Pre-heat the oven to 170°C/325°F/Gas 3. Lay out your slices of beef. Combine the pork sausagemeat, leek and sherry, divide into three and spread each portion over a slice of beef. Roll up each slice and secure with cocktail sticks. Place in a casserole dish. Combine the red wine, beef stock and tomato purée and pour over the beef olives. Cover and cook in the pre-heated oven for 1½ hours, braising the meat occasionally with the cooking liquid.

Chicken apricot olives

Another popular version of beef olives is this recipe, which has always been a great favourite with our two.

3 chicken breasts, skinned and boned
2 tablespoons (30ml) apricot jam
75g (3 oz) pork and apricot sausagemeat (or add some chopped apricot to pork sausagemeat)
glass of white wine (125ml)
125ml (5 fl oz) chicken stock

Pre-heat the oven to 170°C/325°F/Gas 3. Lay out the chicken breasts and tenderise them by bashing a little with a rolling pin. Spread a little apricot jam over each chicken breast and then divide the pork and apricot sausagemeat into three, spreading each portion over a chicken breast. Roll up and secure with cocktail sticks. Place in a casserole dish and pour in the white wine and chicken stock. Cover and cook in the pre-heated oven for 1 hour. Braise occasionally with the cooking liquid.

With both of these dishes if you wish to thicken the cooking liquid you can either add a little cornflour mixed with some cold water to the dish about 20 minutes before the end of the cooking time, or at the end of the cooking time, strain off the juices (leaving the meat olives covered in the oven), bring them to the boil and then cook until the sauce begins to thicken and reduce, then serve over the meat.

Pork and apple slice bake

When you have had a roast lunch you will often have plenty of meat left for the following day. In times gone by this would have been served cold, or minced and made into shepherd's pie or rissoles. I have come up with some very tasty alternatives.

400–600g (1–1½ lb) cold roast pork slices (any fat removed)
3 dessert apples, skinned, cored and sliced
400g (1 lb) potatoes, skinned and thinly sliced
125ml (5 fl oz) single cream
125ml (5 fl oz) milk
knob of butter, melted
1 dessertspoon (10 ml) demerara sugar

Pre-heat the oven to 200°C/400°F/Gas 6. Into a greased shallow oven-proof dish layer the pork, apple and potato slices. Combine the cream and milk and pour onto the bake. Cover with the melted butter and sugar. Cover and cook in the pre-heated oven for 30 minutes. Uncover and cook for a further 20–30 minutes until the top is brown.

Stir-fried lamb and vegetables

This stir fry can, of course, be used for leftover pork, chicken or beef, as well as the lamb that I have used in this recipe.

1 carrot, cut into matchsticks
1 red pepper, core and seeds removed, cut into thin strips
1 tablespoon (15ml) groundnut or sunflower oil
1 courgette, cut into matchsticks
1 leek, halved lengthwise, cleaned and cut into strips
300g (12 oz) cold roast lamb slices, cut into thin strips (remove any fat)
2 tablespoons (30ml) soy or oyster sauce
3 tablespoons (45ml) sherry, white wine, dry vermouth or orange juice
4 tablespoons (60ml) tomato ketchup

Stir fry the carrot and pepper in the oil for two minutes, add the courgette, leek and lamb strips and stir fry for another 2 minutes. Add the remaining ingredients and cook for 1–2 minutes until heated through and the meat and vegetables are coated with the sauce.

Tortilla a la leftovers

You will need a frying pan that will go under the grill, i.e. one with a handle that won't melt.

300g (12 oz) potato, finely cubed
2 tablespoons (30ml) oil
knob of butter
1 onion, diced
1 clove garlic, crushed
100g (4 oz) peas, cooked
100–200g (4–8 oz) leftover roast chicken, pork, etc.,
    cut into small cubes
4 eggs, beaten
sprinkling oregano

Fry the potato in the oil until cooked and brown. If the potato is already cooked this will only take about 2–3 minutes otherwise it will take about 6–8 minutes. Remove the potato from the pan and add the knob of butter and the onion and garlic, cook for a few minutes until softened and just starting to colour. Return the potato to the pan with the peas and meat. Pour in the eggs and oregano. The eggs will quickly begin to set. Cook on a low heat for 2 minutes. Pre-heat the grill. Put the frying pan under the grill and cook until the top of the tortilla is golden brown. Slide onto a plate and cut into wedges to serve.

Finger lickin' chicken

If you have a cool bag or box to transport it in this makes really excellent picnic food as it is easily eaten with the fingers.

2 small chicken breasts (about 450g or 18 oz), skinned and boned
3 tablespoons (45ml) tomato ketchup
1 tablespoon (15ml) soy sauce
1 tablespoon (15ml) wine vinegar
1 tablespoon (15ml) orange juice
3 tablespoons (45ml) water
1 teaspoon (5ml) molasses sugar
oil for greasing

Cut the chicken into strips and place in a bowl. Combine the tomato ketchup, soy sauce, wine vinegar, orange juice and water, pour over the chicken and mix in. Sprinkle with the molasses sugar. Cover and marinade for at least 4 hours or overnight. When ready to cook the chicken, pre-heat the oven to 180°C/350°F/Gas 4. Grease a sheet of baking foil and then transfer the chicken and sauce to the foil. Fold the foil so that the chicken is tightly enclosed and cook in the pre-heated oven for 30 minutes. Then open the foil up and cook for a further 10–15 minutes to brown.

Vicarage roast

This recipe is for any time when you are feeling as 'poor as church mice'. It's delicious with lashings of gravy and vegetables or cold with jacket potatoes. Meatloaves have always been popular in America but have never really caught on here – but do try this recipe as it is very good. This quantity should feed you all twice.

1 small onion, chopped
1 clove garlic, crushed
knob of butter
400g (1 lb) minced lamb, beef or pork
3 slices bread, crumbed
200g (8 oz) sausagemeat (use a good one that is not too fatty)
2 eggs, beaten
1 teaspoon (5ml) Marmite
1 tablespoon (15ml) milk
1 tablespoon (15ml) fresh finely chopped herbs, for example, mint, parsley or sage

Pre-heat the oven to 180°C/350°F/Gas 4. Fry the onion and garlic in the butter until soft and starting to colour. In a separate pan brown the mince and then drain off any fat. Then combine the onions, garlic and mince with the breadcrumbs, sausagemeat, eggs, Marmite, milk and herbs. Put into a greased loaf tin, pressing the mixture in firmly. Bake in the pre-heated oven for 1–1¼ hours until well done – it should be brown on top and a skewer inserted will come out clean. Leave in the tin for 5 minutes before serving.

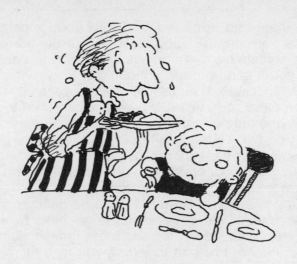

5. Cooking for toddlers

Up until now I have presumed that when you are looking after your children you have generally had to rely on meals that you have prepared and cooked earlier in the day or meals from the freezer, just being able to reheat them at the appropriate time. Certainly this was the case when my two were very young – once they had decided it was lunchtime, it was needed immediately.

However, as they begin to be able to communicate with you and you with them, it is possible to make them understand that mummy (or daddy) is cooking the lunch and that it will be ready soon. As long as this doesn't take very long! So you should have some meals that can be knocked up very quickly – definitely within thirty minutes if your children are like mine.

You should also have some meals that you can quickly knock up just for your children – you may not want to have lunch with them as you intend to eat in the evening and don't want to ruin your appetite, or perhaps you are all eating together but the adults are having something that you know your little ones just won't eat. It can be quite difficult just to cook for your children because their appetites are generally quite small in these early years. It is particularly hard to cater for just one little one, however, if you have very faddy eaters and two children with very different tastes, then this also makes life very difficult.

Often when your child becomes a toddler – and I use this term to cover children from the age of one and above – feeding them can become a lot more difficult. When they were very little it was easier to get them to accept new foods, but as they become more independent and more and more resistant to letting you feed them, they also tend to become a lot more conservative in what they will eat. It is at this stage that a child, who up until now has been a very good eater and not a particular problem to their parents, may become a faddy eater and meal-times can soon disintegrate into a nightmare with the parents trying to get their little darling to eat anything while the toddler is virtually uninterested in any food at all. Helena has still to go through this stage but James certainly ran his mother ragged with periods of complete lack of interest in any food whatever. At one stage he went six weeks hardly eating a thing, and although mother knows that the worst thing you can do is to make an issue of this, it is very hard to remain calm when all the carefully prepared meals you have made are just ending up in the bin. It is amazing just how little they can get away with eating, but if you are really worried you can start giving them vitamin drops. At the end of six weeks I had just given in and got a bottle of these – when James started eating normally again. How do they know!

One thing I did during this phase when he wasn't eating was to give him much more calorific snacks in between meals, such as fruit cake or chocolate, which while being much more sugary and fatty than his normal snacks (fruit, cheese or reduced-sugar biscuits) meant that I was still getting some calories into him. The reason I did this is that under two years old a child will generally achieve half of their adult height and their diet at this age is particularly important. While I was not happy with the balance of James' diet at the time, at least he was still getting some calories, so ensuring that he would not fall too far behind in his growth.

However, it is also important that you don't fall into the trap of giving your child too many fatty or sugary snacks in between meals or they may well be too full up at their proper mealtimes, thereby perpetuating the cycle of them not eating at mealtimes. So if you do want to give your child a nutritious snack make sure that you give it to them at least a couple of hours before their next meal is due. If they are happily eating sandwiches this would be my choice of a good snack, but other good snacks include flapjacks, cheese scones or fruit cake (but make sure that they clean their teeth afterwards). Also be very careful that you are not allowing your toddler to drink too many fluids as this can certainly fill them up.

There really cannot be very many parents who don't worry about what their children are eating at some stage (or not eating to be more particular) so at least you have the comfort of knowing that you are in perfectly good company!

Be very careful about giving your toddler choices at mealtimes – many of them go through an especially infuriating stage when it is virtually impossible for them to make up their minds. You may make a perfectly innocent remark about whether they would like a raspberry or banana yoghurt for tea. They will choose one and immediately change their mind (or worse, wait until you've opened the yoghurt) and this is often accompanied by crying as they really can't decide which they want. Far better at this stage to just present items to them, until they begin to voice strong preferences of their own.

Another aspect of your child's behaviour at this stage may really end up driving you to distraction. Most children will become very inconsistent in their likes and dislikes at this age. For instance, the meal that for the last couple of weeks has been their absolute favourite, that you could always count on them eating all up, may suddenly be greeted by a stony silence and the sight of your toddler just playing with the food on their plate, suddenly taking an inordinate interest in the cat, the fridge, singing songs, trying to slide down from the table (or under the tray of their highchair), anything in fact rather than eating the meal that you have just placed in front of them. When they can talk it becomes even worse as they will remark quite easily that they 'don't like it' and it is of no use whatsoever to try and discuss with them that this is their favourite meal, because once a toddler has decided that they just don't like a meal then you have little chance of getting them to eat it.

One thing that I have never done is to keep a meal that has been rejected and then offer it again, say at teatime. I always throw it straight in the bin, as both of my two are very strong minded and saving it would only result in them not eating anything at teatime as well. However, I do know that some mothers do use this ploy – and it works. If, for instance, your child was just too tired perhaps to eat the meal when it was first offered, after they have had a sleep, they may wolf it down.

There are also some children who can be bribed into eating their savoury course by the promise of a sweet course afterwards. With James I found that if he had to eat something he didn't want to get something he did want then he just wasn't that worried about not getting the sweet. So mother decided that she would rather he ate something rather than nothing at all. Eventually, after a bout of being a faddy eater, he always returns to his normal balanced diet. He's still a little more conservative than mother would like him to be but he does eat a wide variety of foods and I've got plenty of time to bring him round to eating a more exotic diet. I was a real pain to my poor parents. I was into my teens before I really started to develop an interest in food. Prior to that I would eat most meats (but not offal in any form), fishfingers, potato in most of its forms, peas and lots of tomato sauce! So James is already a better eater than I was myself, so I can't really complain!

When you are really looking for quick and easy ways to feed your kids you need to consider whether it is really worth going to the trouble of making 'proper' meals for them. By this I mean a traditional meal of meat and two veg. Many toddlers will be far happier with a toasted snack with a little sweetcorn and tomatoes. I have also found that grated raw vegetables such as carrot or courgette go down well with my two. So don't always feel that you have to put a lot of effort into your cooking. Here are some of the 'toasties' that I have found go down well with my children and their friends. Instead of using bread as a base for your toasties try substituting either crumpets or halved muffins. I have occasionally used plain or cheese scones as well.

Toasties

Cheese toasties
Serves 1

Helena really loves these and enjoys pulling the melted cheese off and sucking it before eating it!

    1 slice bread
    ½ teaspoon (2.5ml) margarine
    25g (1 oz) cheddar or gruyère, grated
    1 teaspoon (5ml) milk

Toast one side of the bread. Combine the margarine, cheese and milk. When the bread has browned, turn it over and fork the cheese mixture onto the untoasted side. Toast again until the cheese has melted and is starting to bubble – don't overcook, most children prefer these less toasted than adults generally prefer them. Cool for 1–2 minutes before cutting off crusts and cutting into squares or triangles for your child. Be very careful when serving these to your children as cheese holds its heat and you certainly don't want your child to burn her mouth.

Sardines on toast
Serves 1

Not all children will eat this recipe for a fish toastie. Again with mine, it is Helena who will eat them but James hates them!

    1 slice wholemeal bread
    1 sardine from a tin of sardines in tomato sauce
    1 dessert spoon (10ml) sauce from tin or tomato
       ketchup
    pinch of fresh finely chopped parsley (optional)

Toast one side of the bread. Mash the sardines (removing bones for very young children – mash them in when your children are older as they are a good source of calcium) with the tomato sauce or ketchup. When the bread has browned, fork the sardine mixture onto the untoasted side, sprinkle with parsley if using and toast for 2 minutes to heat up the sardines. Remove crusts and cut into fingers for your child. Again, be careful not to serve it until it is cool enough for your child.

Pizza toasties
Serves 1

This toastie is nearly universally popular with children and can be varied to incorporate your child's specific likes and dislikes. For example, James loves sweetcorn and some sliced tomatoes added to the topping before cooking it.

> 1 slice of bread
> 2 teaspoons (10ml) tomato ketchup
> 25g (1 oz) cheddar or gruyère cheese, grated
> few celery leaves, finely chopped (optional)

Toast the slice of bread on one side and spread the tomato ketchup on the untoasted side. Sprinkle with the cheese and the finely chopped celery leaves. Toast until the cheese is melting and bubbling.

As well as the sweetcorn and tomato variation I have suggested above, we have found pea and ham to be a good choice (cook the peas before using), and ham and mushrooms is a favourite if your child will eat mushrooms.

Hashes

Although you do not want to give your children too many fried foods there are times when you are really in a hurry when this cooking method is all too easy to resort to – and there is no doubt that many children do like fried foods. However, as frying increases the amount of fat they are getting in their diet do try not to resort to this every day, although it is perfectly okay to fry sometimes. If you do find yourself getting out the frying pan frequently – or worse still it never making it back to the cupboard – then you really need to sit down and rethink how you should be feeding your little monkeys.

After our trip to the United States I found that I started to make many more 'hashes' than I had previously. They are very popular over there and I have found that our children greatly enjoy them. Here are our two favourites. Both will feed two or three children.

Tuna hash

    1 small onion, finely chopped
    ½ small red, green or yellow pepper, diced
    1 tablespoon (15ml) oil
    200g can tuna, drained
    dash Worcestershire sauce
    93g sachet instant mashed potato, made up as directed

Fry the onion and pepper in the oil for 5 minutes. Add the rest of the ingredients and flatten down into the pan to make a potato cake. Cook for 2 minutes and then stir up the mixture, so that the brown bits from the underside are mixed in. Flatten down again and cook for a further 2 minutes. Serve immediately with baked beans or sweetcorn and tomato ketchup.

Corned beef hash

This recipe for hash is a little more authentic than the first and is useful for using up any leftovers from a Sunday roast. I am not a great fan of corned beef but prefer this hash made with corned beef than with leftover beef, which I would rather have in a sandwich or salad.

large knob of butter
1 small onion, finely diced
200g (8 oz) cooked peeled potato, diced
3 tablespoons (45ml) gravy
230g can corned beef, sliced

Melt the butter, add the onion and potato and fry for 5–10 minutes until brown and starting to crisp. Add the gravy and corned beef and mix in well. Fry for a few minutes and then stir again, mixing in the brown crispy underside. Flatten into the pan and cook for a further 2 minutes and then serve.

Pasta

The main ingredient that busy mums resort to time and time again to feed their growing offspring has to be pasta. As a cupboard standby it is hard to beat as it stores easily, comes in many shapes and forms and is a relatively cheap ingredient that cooks in minutes. Therefore I have concocted a number of dishes that use this wonderful ingredient. The amounts will serve two children. (If you are only cooking for one save half and serve it the next day as a bake with some grated cheese and some breadcrumbs on top. For three just increase the amount of pasta and for four double the recipe.)

Penne with creamy salmon sauce

This is a firm favourite on family holidays as there are no special ingredients to buy and it can be whipped up in minutes. It will also keep for another day if we have stopped off on the way home and decided to eat at a local pub or restaurant.

> 50–75g (2–3 oz) penne
> half a small onion, finely chopped
> 1 teaspoon (5ml) butter or oil
> 100g can pink salmon, drained
> small pinch of paprika
> 3–4 tablespoons (45–60ml) double cream
> 1 teaspoon (5ml) tomato ketchup

Cook pasta as directed on packet. Meanwhile fry the onion in the butter or oil until soft, stir in the rest of ingredients and quickly heat through. Serve over drained pasta.

Tuna and green pepper sauce with pasta

50–75g (2–3 oz) pasta
half a green pepper, finely diced
2 teaspoons (10ml) oil
100g can tuna, drained
3–4 tablespoons (45–60ml) double cream

Cook pasta as directed on packet. Meanwhile fry the pepper in the oil until starting to soften and colour (about 5–10 minutes), add the drained tuna and cream and mix well. Heat through to warm up the tuna and serve over the drained pasta.

Chicken with vegetables and pasta

50–75g (2–3 oz) pasta bows
1 ready-cooked chicken breast
1 small courgette, sliced
quarter of a red pepper, finely diced
large knob of butter
squeeze lemon juice

Cook the pasta bows as directed on packet. Take the skin and any bone off the ready-cooked chicken and shred the meat into bite-sized pieces. Gently cook the courgette and pepper in the butter for 5 minutes until just beginning to brown. Add the lemon juice. Drain the pasta bows and serve with the chicken, vegetables and buttery juices all mixed in.

Tagliatelle with ham and peas

50–75g (2–3 oz) tagliatelle
50g (2 oz) peas
50g (2 oz) thinly sliced ham
large knob of butter or 2–3 tablespoons (30–45ml)
    double cream

Cook the tagliatelle as directed on the packet. Either cook the peas in a separate pan or add to the cooking tagliatelle (depending on what size pan you have to cook in). When the pasta is cooked, drain it and add the rest of the ingredients, gently heat through and serve immediately.

Spaghetti with mushrooms and herbs

If your children like mushrooms they will love this recipe. I sometimes add some peas to it as well.

50–75g (2–3 oz) spaghetti
100g (4 oz) mushrooms, sliced
25g (1 oz) unsalted butter
1 tablespoon (15ml) chopped fresh parsley or a little
    less of chopped fresh sage
shavings of cheddar or gruyère cheese to serve

Cook the spaghetti as directed on the packet. Meanwhile cook the mushrooms in the butter until soft, stir in the herbs and serve over the cooked, drained spaghetti. Top with some shavings of cheddar or gruyère cheese.

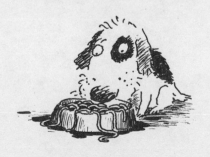

Spaghetti with bacon and cream

This is also very good if you have any hard boiled eggs to hand which you can shell, chop roughly and add at the last minute. Also if you have some, and can be bothered, skinned, chopped cherry tomatoes are wonderful added to this dish at the last minute.

50–75g (2–3 oz) spaghetti
2–3 slices of streaky or back bacon
3–4 tablespoons (45–60ml) double cream

Cook the spaghetti as directed on the packet. Meanwhile grill the bacon to suit your child's requirements (but the crispier the better, as this removes the most fat). When the bacon is cooked cut into bite-sized pieces. Drain the spaghetti when cooked and add the bacon and cream and heat through gently before serving.

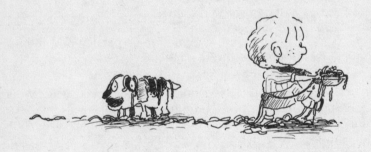

Pasta with courgettes and butter beans

  50–75g (2–3 oz) pasta bows
  1 small courgette, sliced
  large knob of butter
  200g can butter beans, drained
  3–4 tablespoons (45–60ml) double cream
  50g (2 oz) grated cheddar or gruyère cheese
  sprinkling chopped fresh sage

Cook the pasta bows as directed on the packet. Meanwhile gently fry the courgette in the butter until just starting to brown (about 5 minutes), add the butter beans and cream and heat through gently. Drain the pasta. Just before serving, stir the cheese and sage into the other ingredients, then just as it is starting to melt mix these ingredients into your cooked, drained pasta bows.

Pasta spirals with tomato sauce

  50–75g (2–3 oz) pasta spirals
  half a small onion, finely chopped
  knob of butter
  200g can chopped tomatoes
  4 tomatoes, skinned and chopped
  1 dessertspoon (10ml) tomato purée
  sprinkling chopped fresh parsley to serve
  shavings of cheddar or gruyère cheese to serve

Cook the pasta spirals as directed on the packet. Meanwhile gently fry the onion in the melted butter until starting to soften (about 5 minutes), add the can of chopped tomatoes, the fresh skinned and chopped tomatoes and the tomato purée and gently simmer for a few minutes. When the pasta is cooked, drain and serve topped with the tomato sauce and the parsley and shavings of cheese.

Breakfast pasta

If you find yourself with some leftovers from a cooked breakfast, cover them and refrigerate and then you will be able to make this easy pasta dish for the children, not to eat at breakfast – but then you never know with kids . . .

50–75g (2–3 oz) pasta spirals or bows
half a small onion, finely chopped
1 teaspoon (5ml) oil
200g can chopped tomatoes
1–2 cooked sausages, thinly sliced
1–2 slices pre-cooked bacon, cut into bite-sized strips

Cook the pasta spirals or bows as directed on the packet. Gently fry the onion in the oil until just starting to soften and colour (about 5 minutes), then add the chopped tomatoes and cook for a few more minutes. Just before serving add the sausage and bacon and heat through before serving on the cooked, drained pasta.

Banana and peanut butter pasta

This recipe seems a very strange invention but it has proved to be very popular with children. It is a variation of a pasta dish that I first devised for students (who are generally very open minded about what they will eat).

50–75g (2–3 oz) pasta bows
1 tablespoon (15ml) soft margarine or melted butter
1 tablespoon (15ml) milk
1 tablespoon (15ml) smooth peanut butter
1 ripe banana, mashed

Cook the pasta bows as directed on packet. Meanwhile blend together the margarine or butter, milk and peanut butter, than mix in with the mashed banana. When the pasta is cooked, drain and mix with the banana butter. Heat through very gently and serve.

Convenience foods

When you are in a particular hurry to feed your child you may often resort to some form of convenience food. As long as these are not all you are feeding your child there is no reason why you should not occasionally resort to them. The main problem with convenience foods (and this goes for most adult meals as well) is that they are generally higher in sugar and salt than is recommended for us. Many are often lower in nutritional value than we would want as well. Therefore I have concocted a few meals using some common convenience foods that I hope go some way to remedying these deficiencies.

Cheese and tomato pizza

Although a manufactured cheese and tomato pizza will be higher in fat and salt than is generally recommended it does provide a good range of vitamins and minerals. To make into a complete meal for a toddler, add some pre-cooked sliced chicken to the topping and serve with some extra vegetables (a salad – if your child likes this – of grated carrot, courgette and sliced banana or orange segments goes well, or some cooked carrot and broccoli).

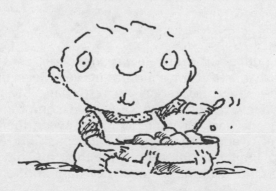

Baked beans

Again even if using the reduced salt and sugar varieties – which I thoroughly recommend for youngsters – the level of these will still be higher than is desirable. However, they are a great convenience food served with either bread or toast (I have found that both of my two are very keen on walnut bread and will eat it unbuttered, thereby cutting their fat consumption). I also serve a few sliced tomatoes with baked beans and if you serve this meal with a drink of fresh orange juice or follow it with an orange, you improve its nutritional value as the iron in the beans is more easily absorbed when vitamin C is present – especially important for vegetarian children as it helps the body to absorb iron from vegetable sources.

Burgers

Many children adore burgers and if they are 100 per cent meat and are grilled then they are not the baddies that they are often made out to be as they are a good source of protein and iron. Serve with a bap (not chips as this makes a meal with a very high fat content) and again either a salad or some vegetables – peas or sweetcorn and tomatoes are extremely quick to prepare and very good for children.

Oven chips

When opting for chips (everyone deserves an occasional treat, and most children are very keen on chips) try to serve the thicker-style oven chips. My children unfortunately detest these so I have compromised by serving one pack of micro chips between them – you only get twenty-four chips in each pack and so I am able to limit the amount of fat they are having. Try serving chips with baked beans or ham and tomatoes.

Fish fingers

With these it is important to choose a brand which is made from whole fish fillets. Don't be surprised if the fish is not cod or haddock – the ones that we use are actually pollack. The nutritional value is higher when whole fish are used rather than fish trimmings which tend to have cereals added. Another reason for opting for a brand that uses whole fish fillets is that they taste much better – they may be more expensive but they are well worth it. Fish fingers provide a good source of protein, vitamins and minerals – and in many cases is the only fish that children will eat (even if you have to cover them in tomato sauce to get them to eat them). Always grill or oven bake – don't fry as you will then be adding a disproportionate amount of fat to the meal, lowering its overall nutritional value. Serve with salad and tasty bread or some cooked vegetables – broccoli and sweetcorn are favourites in our house.

Chicken nuggets

Pieces of chicken coated in breadcrumbs can be bought either frozen or chilled. They can also be found in many different shapes and forms, masquerading as feet, dinosaurs, etc. Although these may occasionally encourage children to try a food that they would not normally eat, I cannot recommend these ranges. I have only bought chicken nuggets when I have found them made from whole pieces of chicken breast, and these are few and far between. Mostly they will be made from reformed meat which may contain only 30–50 per cent meat. The other drawback is that the more breadcrumb coating that you have in relation to meat then the lower the nutritional value of the nugget. Again oven baking is recommended as frying will not help to make chicken nuggets healthy food. However, if these guidelines are borne in mind when choosing your product then they are a good source of protein, vitamins and minerals.

Serve with tasty bread, salad or vegetables – or baked beans as the salt content of chicken nuggets is fairly low.

By the way, one of James' little friends went through a phase when she would only eat chicken nuggets for her lunch. This went on for quite a long time, and it certainly hasn't adversely affected her. So don't worry if your child does sometimes develop an obsession for one type of food – they will eventually grow out of it!

Fruit, vegetables and cereals

These are the very best types of convenience foods. Whenever you are really in a hurry and have absolutely no time to feed your child at all – this generally happens when you have an appointment to keep and you have tried to accommodate your child's sudden need for a sleep – then you can always resort to apples, pears and bananas. If you have a little more time then you can throw together a quick meal using slices of ripe avocado mixed with tomatoes and canned sweetcorn. Many children will eat this very happily with some bread.

Whenever I am really desperate for time and have no chance to cook at all then I give my children some tasty bread. There are many lovely ones on the market now that are part-baked. I take them home, bake them and then divide them up and freeze them. They don't take long to defrost and I can have children-sized portions without wasting the rest of the loaf. Otherwise choose from the selection of rolls that are available individually; these are much tastier than normal sliced loaves. Serve with some thin slices of cheese (or grated if this is what your child prefers) and open a can of sweetcorn, slice some tomatoes and add some grated carrot and you have a great child-friendly meal. Follow with some sliced banana and halved grapes. This meal is also very adaptable and transports easily so makes a great basis for a picnic.

As an alternative to the cheese, try your child on some canned chick peas or kidney beans – many children do enjoy these. As an anytime snack give your child some dry cereal – I have found Cheerios to be very popular. Muesli (of the no-added-sugar variety) goes down well mixed with yoghurt. Most children will eat hot oat cereals and you can add to their nutritional value by serving with slices of banana, strawberries, raisins or grapes. Cereals can come in very handy as most are fortified with iron and vitamins but just try to avoid the varieties with masses of added sugar.

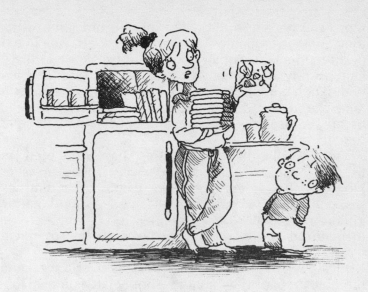

6. Batch cooking

There are many times when we just don't have time to cook. With both of my children we have always had very busy mornings – toddler groups, tumble tots, swimming and visiting the crèche while mother gets some exercise (and a respite from them)! So when we have rushed back from our morning activity it is usually too late to start cooking. Therefore I have tended to do a lot of batch cooking, dividing dishes into child-sized portions and freezing for use at a later date. I usually include some vegetables in these dishes but try to serve some fresh veggies with them as well, which I normally prepare at breakfast time and reheat later. This is not ideal – if you can, persuade your children that they don't have to eat the moment they walk through the door as it is better to cook your veggies then.

We often have baked potatoes with our lunch as

these can be put in the oven and the timer set so that they are ready when we appear. If we are having rice or pasta then again mother cooks it at breakfast so that it can be reheated when we return. The only problem with batch cooking is that you do need to remember to take the required dish out of the freezer the night before, or else it will be baked potatoes with cheese for lunch!

Virtually all of the dishes in this chapter are tried and trusted family meals that we have cooked for ages. However, I have compromised a little by adding less seasoning than we used to use as I have found that my children generally prefer plainer food – roll on the teenage years when we can return to lots of spicier food.

I usually cook some of these dishes over a weekend, thereby preparing a month's supply at a time. Don't forget to wrap them properly in freezer bags or foil tins and label the contents and the date you made them. It's amazing how alike many dishes look when they're frozen. (I get all of my freezer bags, ties, etc. from Lakeland Plastics – I use a lot of their boil-a-bags, which can be used in the freezer and the microwave, as well as heated in boiling water.)

Because both of my children have small appetites – and even mother doesn't like a large helping at lunch-time – one casserole goes a long way. So most of these casseroles will make between four and six meals. I try to give some indication of how many meals you should get but of course this will depend on your child's appetite. For instance, Delyth, one of James' friends, has been able to eat a whole pork chop since she was two years old, while one pork chop still feeds James and Helena easily. So in this chapter one meal is the amount I would use roughly to serve one small adult portion and two children. (My husband would eat the entire amount himself!) I don't like to keep food for too long in the freezer and never cook more than I would use up in two months. So in one weekend I can easily make enough batches to feed us for the coming month.

Once you have made the dish, cool quickly and divide into portions that will suit your family. You can either cut the meat into bite-sized pieces or leave until reheated and served. The latter option is usually preferable as freezing can have a drying effect on food and it is generally better to leave the meat in bigger portions and to cut it up to suit your children when serving.

Mince
Makes 4–8 meals

One of the most common dishes served to children is mince in one of its many forms so I often make up a big batch. Here I use extra lean mince; if you use ordinary mince you will get a lot of fat released when frying – tip this out before continuing with the recipe or the resulting dish will be too fatty. I now cook mince with beef or half beef and half pork, but I have also made it with lamb and venison and it is always popular with the children whatever meat I have used. My mince has a strong tomato flavour; you can use less tomato purée and add a crumbled Oxo cube for a more traditional flavour if you wish.

    1 large onion, chopped
    1 garlic clove, crushed
    1–2 large carrots, finely diced
    2–3 tablespoons (30–45ml) olive oil
    900g (2 lb) of minced beef or a mixture of beef and
        pork
    200g tube tomato purée
    400g can chopped tomatoes
    1 red pepper, core and seeds removed and flesh diced
    1 tablespoon (15ml) Worcestershire sauce
    sprinkling of thyme

Pre-heat the oven to 150°C/300°F/Gas 2. Gently fry the onion, garlic and carrot in the oil until just soft and starting to colour (approximately 5–10 minutes). Remove to a large casserole dish. Place the mince in your frying pan and cook until the meat has browned. Keep stirring to break up any lumps. Now add the tomato purée and stir in. Add the rest of the ingredients and 250ml (10 fl oz) of water (I do sometimes add red wine, it improves the flavour and the alcohol cooks off). Stir and bring to a simmer. Now add everything to the casserole dish, cover and place in the oven for 2 hours. Remove the lid, stir and cook for a further 30 minutes. Use as a basis for spaghetti sauce or for shepherd's pie or just serve with baked potatoes.

Lasagne
Makes 2–4 meals

I often use half of the mince from the preceding recipe to make this lasagne.

> half of the cooked mince from preceding recipe
> 500ml (1 pint) of cheese sauce (see page 97)
> 8 sheets of no-cook lasagne
> 50g (2 oz) cheese, grated

Pre-heat the oven to 180°C/350°F/Gas 4. In a large shallow oven-proof dish, spread 2 tablespoons of the mince mixture, cover with half of the lasagne sheets and half of the cheese sauce. Spoon the rest of the mince on top and cover with the remaining lasagne. Top with the rest of the cheese sauce and sprinkle with cheese. Cook in the pre-heated oven for 30–45 minutes until brown on top.

This recipe for lasagne can also be used to make a vegetarian lasagne. For this, omit the meat mince and substitute ratatouille (see page 158) or use a soya mince for the filling. You can also make lasagnes with most cooked vegetable fillings or a mixture of fish and vegetables. You may be more successful at getting your children to eat vegetables such as spinach if you mix them into a lasagne with other vegetables that they like.

Meatballs
Makes 3–4 meals

I usually serve meatballs with rice but do sometimes serve with tagliatelle or even with Chinese egg noodles.

> 2 slices wholemeal bread, crusts removed and crumbed
> 2 tablespoons (30ml) milk or 1 egg, beaten
> 500g (1 lb) lean, ground beef
> 1 tablespoon (15ml) fresh chopped parsley
> 1–2 tablespoons (15–30ml) olive oil
>
> *Sauce*
> 2 × 400g cans of chopped tomatoes
> 1 tablespoon (15ml) tomato purée
> 250ml (10 fl oz) water or red wine
> sprinkling of oregano

Place the breadcrumbs, milk or egg, beef and parsley in a food processor and combine (alternatively, place in a large bowl and mix well). Take the resulting ball and divide into 6 equal portions. Divide each portion into 5 and using your hands roll into little balls (this is easier if you flour your hands first) so you end up with 30 little meatballs. In a large pan heat the oil (you need a thin layer over the bottom of the pan) and fry the meatballs (it is generally easier to do this a few at a time). When brown all over return all the meatballs to the pan and add the sauce ingredients. Cover and simmer for 20–30 minutes until the meatballs are cooked through.

Lamb casserole
Makes 4–6 meals

900g (2 lb) braising or casserole lamb, cubed
2 carrots, diced
1 onion, diced
2 sticks of celery, sliced, including the celery leaves
(they improve the flavour)
1 bayleaf
sprinkling of thyme or mint
375ml (15 fl oz) lamb stock or water

You will need a casserole dish that can be used on the hob as well as in the oven. Pre-heat the oven to 170°C/325°F/Gas 3. Place all the ingredients in the casserole dish, and on the hob bring up to a simmer. Cover, place in the oven and cook for 1½ hours. Then strain the cooking liquid into a saucepan and boil until reduced by half. Remove the bayleaf and mix in the cooking liquid. Divide into portions and freeze. When serving I sometimes add a little crème fraîche or cream when reheating the casserole.

Chicken casserole
Makes 2–4 meals

1 onion, sliced
1 clove garlic, crushed
1 carrot, sliced
1 stick of celery, sliced
1 tablespoon (15ml) olive oil
4 chicken breasts, boned and skinned
375ml (15 fl oz) chicken stock or water
1 bayleaf
2 tablespoons (30ml) butter
3 tablespoons (45ml) flour

Pre-heat the oven to 180°C/350°F/Gas 4. Gently fry the onion, garlic, carrot and celery in the oil until just starting to soften and colour (approximately 5–10 minutes). Place in a casserole dish and add the chicken breasts, stock or water and the bayleaf. Cover and cook for 1 hour. Blend together the butter and flour. Take out the casserole and put on a medium heat on the hob. Gradually add a little of the mixed flour and butter mixture, stirring all the time, and the sauce will gradually thicken. When you have a consistency that you like, you can cool the casserole.

Chicken Marengo
Makes 2–4 meals

This recipe for chicken Marengo is not as authentic as it should be as my two are not keen on mushrooms so I have omitted them and I have also substituted sherry for the wine. If your children are keen on mushrooms you can add some fried in butter to the finished dish.

   4 chicken breasts, boned and skinned
   2 tablespoons (30ml) olive oil
   1 onion, diced
   2 carrots, diced
   1 stick of celery, including leaves, sliced
   1 bouquet garni
   400g can chopped tomatoes
   250ml (10 fl oz) chicken stock or water
   2 tablespoons (30ml) medium dry sherry or orange
      juice
   sprinkling of chopped parsley

Pre-heat the oven to 180°C/350°F/Gas 4. Fry the chicken until brown in half of the oil and then place in a casserole dish. Now in the rest of the oil gently fry the onion, carrot and celery until starting to soften and colour (about 5–10 minutes). Add to the casserole with the bouquet garni, tomatoes, stock or water and sherry or orange juice. Cover and cook for 1 hour. Remove the chicken breasts and discard the bouquet garni, then blend or mouli the remaining ingredients. (Personally I prefer to put it through the mouli – it takes a little longer to do but I prefer the resulting sauce.) Divide the sauce between the chicken pieces. Sprinkle with parsley.

Cod in sauce
Makes 4–6 meals

1.5kg (3½lb) chunky cod fillets
2 carrots, diced
200g can sweetcorn
750ml (1½ pints) milk
3 tablespoons (45ml) cornflour

Place the cod fillets in a saucepan and cover with water. Bring to the boil and then simmer until cooked (about 15 minutes). When cooked, drain and check for and remove any bones and discard any skin. Meanwhile cook the carrots until tender (about 10 minutes) and drain the sweetcorn. Blend 125ml (5 fl oz) of the milk with the cornflour. Put the remaining milk in a small saucepan and bring to the boil, then simmer while adding the cornflour mixture, stirring until it thickens. Pour over the fish and add the carrots and sweetcorn. Mix.

Lamb and barley casserole
Makes 1–2 meals

1 onion, chopped
1 carrot, chopped
1 turnip, chopped
1 tablespoon (15ml) sunflower oil
300g (12 oz) extra lean casserole lamb
50g (2 oz) pearl barley
1 tablespoon (15ml) chopped fresh parsley
1 teaspoon (5ml) cornflour

Pre-heat the oven to 170°C/325°F/Gas 3. Quickly fry the onion, carrot and turnip in the oil until just starting to soften. Add the lamb and brown. Transfer to a casserole dish and add the pearl barley and the parsley, mix well. Just cover with boiling water, put the casserole lid on and cook in the pre-heated oven for 1½ hours. Then, 30 minutes before the cooking time is up, mix the cornflour with a little water and stir into the casserole.

Lamb Provence
Makes 4–8 meals

This recipe is ideal if you want a change from a beef mince dish. I cooked this up during the summer when the BSE scare was at its height and lovely seasonal vegetables were bountiful.

Although James is usually not a great lover of aubergine for some reason he will happily eat it in this dish. I have tried varying the recipe by using grilled slices of aubergine and sometimes frying the aubergine first, but in these cases he never eats it. I have also tried making it with chickpeas and some fresh mint, which Helena thought was lovely but once again James thought was disgusting. It is very difficult to introduce new dishes when one of your guinea pigs is so definite in his likes and dislikes!

> 1 onion, chopped
> 2 cloves garlic, crushed
> 1 carrot, diced
> 1 red pepper, core removed, seeded and diced
> 2 tablespoons (30ml) olive oil
> 900g (2 lb) minced lamb
> 450g (1lb) tomatoes, skinned and chopped, or 400g
>   can chopped tomatoes
> 1 medium aubergine or 2 courgettes, diced
> 2 tablespoons (30ml) tomato purée
> 375ml (15 fl oz) lamb stock or red wine and water
> sprinkling of herbes de Provence or fresh chopped
>   basil

Fry the onion, garlic, carrot and pepper in the oil until starting to soften and colour (about 5–10 minutes). Remove to a plate and fry the minced lamb until browned, stirring to break up lumps. Now return the vegetables to the dish and add the rest of the ingredients. Bring to the boil and then cover and simmer for 30 minutes. Delicious on pasta but also very good with crusty bread.

Chicken with honey and orange
Makes 4–8 meals

Chicken is generally popular with children and I have found that braised chicken has been the most acceptable when they are very young. I have made this and the next one with both free-range chickens and guinea fowl and both were greeted with appreciation.

1.5kg (3½lb) chicken (or guinea fowl)
50g (2 oz) unsalted butter
125ml (5 fl oz) white wine or chicken stock
125ml (5 fl oz) orange juice
3 tablespoons (45ml) runny honey
2 tablespoons (30ml) boiling water
2 oranges

Pre-heat the oven to 180°C/350°F/Gas 4. Put the chicken in a large oven-proof casserole dish. Dot with the butter, and add the white wine or stock and the orange juice to the dish. Cover and cook in the oven for 1 hour. When the hour is up take the casserole dish out of the oven, mix the honey and boiling water and pour over the chicken. Return to the oven without covering and cook for a further 30 minutes. When cooking time is up remove the chicken and strain the cooking sauce into a saucepan. Bring to the boil and reduce by about a third. Take as much meat off the chicken as possible and divide into portions. Peel the orange and divide into segments, removing any pips. Divide the segments and the sauce between the portions of meat and freeze.

Chicken in a pot
Makes 4–8 meals

1 onion, chopped
1 carrot, sliced
50g (2 oz) unsalted butter
1.5kg (3½lb) chicken
1 bouquet garni
sprinkling of thyme or parsley
150ml (10 fl oz) chicken stock or dry white wine

Pre-heat the oven to 190°C/375°F/Gas 5. Place the onion and carrot in the bottom of a large casserole dish. Put a little of the butter inside the chicken and place on the vegetables. Dot the chicken with the rest of the butter. Place the bouquet garni in among the vegetables and sprinkle the thyme or parsley into the stock or wine and then pour this over the chicken. Cover and cook for 1½ hours. If you would like a crispy skin on your chicken uncover for the last 30 minutes of cooking. Cool, divide into portions and freeze.

Pot-roasted beef
Makes 4–8 meals

Although we don't tend to serve up beef very often in our household there is one dish that is very popular – pot-roasted beef. This is probably due to the very long cooking time which produces meat which is meltingly tender. And I do know that in a couple of our friends' house (Ray and Sarah's, whose children are six, three and one) this is the outstanding choice for their Sunday lunch.

> 1 tablespoon (15ml) groundnut or sunflower oil
> 1.5kg (3½lb) boned and rolled brisket of beef
> 1 potato, peeled and sliced
> 1 turnip, peeled and sliced
> 2 carrots, peeled and sliced
> 1 onion, chopped
> 375ml (15 fl oz) beef stock
> pinch of dry mustard
> 1 garlic clove, crushed
> dash of Worcestershire sauce

Pre-heat the oven to 170°C/325°F/Gas 3. Heat the oil in a large frying pan and quickly brown the meat in this. Put the vegetables in the bottom of a large casserole dish. Place the browned beef on these. Mix the stock with the dry mustard powder, garlic and the Worcestershire sauce. Pour over the beef. Cover and cook in the pre-heated oven for at least 3 hours and preferably 3½. Remove the meat and vegetables and strain the cooking liquid into a saucepan, bring to the boil and reduce by about a third before dividing it up with the meat and vegetables and freezing.

Pork Seville
Makes 2–4 meals

1 onion, chopped
knob of butter
4 pork chops
250ml (10 fl oz) orange juice
3 tablespoons (45ml) medium dry sherry (or increase
orange juice)

Pre-heat the oven to 180°C/350°F/Gas 4. Cook the onion in the butter until soft and starting to brown (about 5–10 minutes). Place in the bottom of a shallow oven-proof dish. Lay the pork chops in a single layer over the onion. Pour in the orange juice and sherry if using. Cover and cook in the pre-heated oven for 1 hour. Remove the pork chops and then blend or mouli the onions and the cooking liquid. Divide into portions and freeze.

Sweetened pork with pineapple
Makes 2–4 meals

4 pork chops
230g can pineapple rings in juice
1 tablespoon (15ml) brown sugar

Pre-heat the oven to 180°C/350°F/Gas 4. Place the pork chops in the bottom of an oven-proof dish and add the juice from the canned pineapple. Cover and cook for 45 minutes. Place a pineapple ring on each chop and sprinkle with the brown sugar. Return uncovered to the oven and cook for a further 5–10 minutes, just to melt the sugar. Divide into portions and freeze.

Sausage casserole
Makes 2–4 meals

There are many different types of sausages on the market now and although you can make this quick casserole with ordinary pork sausages, I like to ring the changes by using different types. Our favourites have been pork and leek, pork and apple, beef and tomato, Lincolnshire and Cumberland sausages. It was also well received when I made it with local venison sausages. Just remember that the better the sausage that is used (i.e. with a high meat content) the better the resulting casserole will be.

450g (1 lb) sausages
1 tablespoon (15ml) oil
450g (1 lb) dessert apples, peeled, cored and sliced
    into thick chunks
1 green pepper, cored and finely diced
400g can chopped tomatoes
125ml (5 fl oz) cider or apple juice
dash of Worcestershire sauce

Pre-heat the oven to 190°C/375°F/Gas 5. Fry the sausages in the oil until brown on all sides. Place all the ingredients in a large casserole dish, cover and cook in the oven for 1¼ hours.

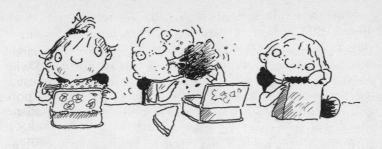

7. Vegetarian meals

Although, of course, a lot of the recipes in this book are vegetarian I thought that we should have a chapter on vegetarian meals as so many children are now being brought up in vegetarian households. However, this chapter is not just for those who only follow a vegetarian diet. It has become increasingly obvious that many people in this country still do not include enough vegetables in their diet, and that in numerous ways this contributes to many types of illness being more prevalent in this country. We should all be aiming for at least a couple of vegetarian meals in our weekly diet and if our children are brought up in this fashion then hopefully it will be second nature to them when they one day have to plan their own meals.

However, alongside this growth of vegetarianism in children, there has also been an increase in the lack of iron in children's diets. This is not to say that by having a vegetarian diet a child will necessarily be lacking in this essential mineral, just that certain guidelines should be followed to ensure that your child does get enough of this particular mineral, and in truth it is more likely to be parents who are not vegetarians themselves who are not aware of these guidelines and are therefore unwittingly not following them.

The most important factor to remember is quite simply that although some vegetables are good sources of iron in the diet it is not as easily digested as iron from meat sources. However, this is easily remedied by ensuring that a good source of vitamin C is also taken at the same time as this helps the body to absorb the iron. With small children who only have small appetites, often the best way of giving them this vitamin C is through a fruit juice – two that are particularly high in vitamin C are orange juice and blackcurrant juice, but do ensure that you give them the unsweetened or 'lite' versions (and compare makes; this can be difficult to do but when I compared a store own-brand version with Ribena, I found that the store version had half as much sugar again as Ribena). Some squashes are also fortified with vitamin C. Other good food sources are tomatoes and broccoli, but bear in mind that this vitamin can be destroyed by overcooking.

Another important point to bear in mind about veg-etarian meals is that they are often high in fibre. Now although in an adult diet this is a benefit it can be more problematical in children. The under fives need a high-energy diet but often they have very small appe-tites. Therefore a meal that is particularly high in fibre may well result in filling them up before their energy needs have been fulfilled. Don't make the mistake of thinking that fibre is a bad thing in itself for children – it is highly beneficial to our digestive systems and hope-fully your children will gradually move to a high-fibre diet as they grow up, thereby lessening their chances of diet-related problems in later life. It is the effect of too much fibre at this young age that is the problem. One other point is that too much fibre in the diet will interfere with the absorption of other essential minerals such as calcium and zinc. So an energy-rich, low-fibre diet is important in the under fives but even more so in the under twos.

As long as your child is having a variety of dairy

foods as well as a variety of plant foods, they should not have any problems. The easiest way to ensure that those who do not eat meat (which is a good source of iron in the diet) are getting enough iron is to give a piece of fruit or a green leafy vegetable with the meal because vitamin C helps the absorption of iron from plant tissues. I also favour freshly squeezed orange juice or blackcurrant juice as a drink with the meal (but not in between meals as these are high in fruit sugars which can lead to damage to the teeth – better to give them as part of a meal).

As long as you are aware of these factors and take care in planning your vegetarian meals there is no reason for your child not to have a perfectly balanced diet (as much as any child has a perfectly balanced diet!). Remember that in ensuring your child has some vegetarian meals in their diet you are helping them along the path to a healthy balanced diet.

In this chapter I have indicated approximately how many meals each recipe should give you; roughly I count one meal as enough to feed a parent and two children or two parents. Therefore if I indicate three meals this should feed mum (or dad) and two kids for lunch two days running and feed mum and dad for one supper. As always this is dependent on your own family (its make up and appetites). I have also indicated meals which are not really suitable for children under one year old with an asterisk (*), either because of the salt content or because I feel that the fibre content is not particularly suitable for the very young.

Cheese and lentil bake*
Makes 2–3 meals

Lentils are a very high-fibre food so only serve this in small quantities. I like to serve it with tomatoes and broccoli. James like tomato ketchup with his while I have managed to get Helena to enjoy hers with a sauce made from natural yoghurt with a little chopped fresh parsley mixed in.

1 onion, chopped
1 clove garlic, crushed
1 tablespoon (15ml) olive, groundnut or sunflower oil
200g (8 oz) red split lentils
500ml (1 pint) vegetable stock
2 carrots, finely grated
8 tablespoons (120ml) cooked rice
1 teaspoon (5ml) Marmite
1 egg, beaten
50g (2 oz) grated cheddar cheese

Topping
3–4 tomatoes, sliced
50g (2 oz) grated cheddar cheese

Pre-heat the oven to 190°C/375°F/Gas 5. Fry the onion and garlic in the oil until starting to soften and colour (about 5–10 minutes). Add the lentils and stock and cook gently until all of the stock is absorbed. Remove from the heat and stir in the remaining ingredients. Put into an 18 × 28cm (7 × 11 in) baking tin which you have lined with baking paper. Cook in the pre-heated oven for 15 minutes until just firm to the touch. Place the sliced tomatoes and grated cheese on top and cook for a further 15 minutes. This bake will keep for a couple of days in the fridge if well covered. So this amount usually feeds mum and two children for two lunches and one evening meal for mum and dad.

Apple veggie pie
Makes 1–2 meals

I have found that many ideas that I first thought up for students have stood me in good stead when it has come to devising dishes for my children – this is because both students and children don't have the same reservations as many people as to what ingredients can be mixed with others! This next dish is a variant on a pie that I first thought up as a student dish. My kids adore it. This should make a lunch for mum and two kids with some leftovers as a side dish for the evening meal.

> half a small onion, chopped
> 1 carrot, diced
> 1 tablespoon (15ml) groundnut or sunflower oil
> 50g (2 oz) broccoli florets, chopped
> 2 dessert apples, cored, peeled and cut into chunks
> 2 tablespoons (30ml) sweetcorn
> 250ml (10 fl oz) cheese sauce (see page 97)
> 1 slice white bread, crumbed
> 2 tablespoons (30ml) mayonnaise
> 50g (2 oz) grated cheddar cheese

Pre-heat the oven to 180°C/350°F/Gas 4. Quickly fry the onion and carrot in the oil until starting to soften (about 5 minutes). Add the broccoli and apple and stir fry for 2 minutes. Put the apples and the fried veggies in a pie dish or gratin dish. Mix in the sweetcorn and the cheese sauce. Mix together the breadcrumbs, mayonnaise and the cheese and spoon over the apple and veggie mixture. Bake in the pre-heated oven for 25–30 minutes until browning. For younger children this will make a complete meal just served with a fruit juice, for older children serve with sliced tomatoes or carrot fingers.

Apple and veg stir fry
Makes 1 meal

half a red pepper, diced
few green beans, mangetout or sugar snap peas
2 tablespoons (30ml) sweetcorn kernels
2 dessert apples, cored, peeled and cut into slices
1 tablespoon (15ml) groundnut oil
1 tablespoon (15ml) apple juice
1 teaspoon (5ml) soy sauce – you can use up to a
   tablespoon if your children like this
1 teaspoon (5ml) tomato ketchup

Quickly fry the vegetables and apple in the oil for 2–3 minutes until starting to soften. Add the apple juice, soy sauce and tomato ketchup and continue to stir fry for another 2 minutes. Serve with rice and a fruit juice.

Mushroom pâté
Makes 1–2 meals

200g (8 oz) chestnut mushrooms, chopped
half a small onion, finely chopped
50g (2 oz) unsalted butter
2 tablespoons (30ml) medium dry sherry
tiny, tiny pinch of nutmeg

Gently fry the mushrooms and onion in half of the butter until very soft. Add the sherry and continue cooking until all of the liquid has evaporated. Cool and then blend with the rest of the butter and season carefully. Use as a topping for crackers or French bread, or use it to fill little vol-au-vents or pastry shells. Mix with a little Greek yoghurt to use as a dip for fresh vegetables. I have found it to be very popular with children (and adults as well).

Cheese topped vegetable crumble
Makes 1–2 meals

2 carrots, diced
100g (4 oz) broccoli florets, sliced
4 tablespoons (120ml) sweetcorn kernels
3 plum tomatoes, skinned and cut into quarters
100g (4 oz) new potatoes, cooked and sliced
125ml (5 fl oz) cheese sauce (see page 97)
sprinkling chopped fresh parsley (optional)
1 tablespoon (15ml) butter
2 tablespoons (30ml) plain flour
1 tablespoon (15ml) porridge oats
50g (2 oz) grated gruyère or cheddar cheese

Pre-heat the oven to 190°C/375°F/Gas 5. Cook the carrots for 8 minutes in boiling water, steaming the broccoli above them. When cooked mix with the sweetcorn kernels, the plum tomatoes and the potatoes. Mix the vegetables with the cheese sauce and place in a pie or gratin dish. Sprinkle with the parsley if using. Rub the butter and flour together using your fingertips until the mixture resembles breadcrumbs. Mix in the oats and cheese and use as a topping for the vegetables. Bake in the pre-heated oven for 25–30 minutes until starting to brown on top. This really needs no accompaniment apart from a fruit juice unless you wish to serve a small salad with it (then my choice would be a watercress and orange salad, or some plain sliced tomatoes).

Mock bobotie
Makes 1–2 meals

Unusually for me this is a cookery book that has very few recipes for curries or other 'spicy' foods. Quite simply I have found that my two children are not very keen on them – which I find very ironic! However, we do know from our friends that not all children have this strange aversion to spicy foods. Only this week our friend Sarah was telling me about how much their four-year-old had enjoyed grandad's spicy chilli at the weekend. So we can only hope that ours will gradually grow into liking spicy foods and I do occasionally try them on a very mildly spiced dish – this is one that has met with some approval.

1 slice white bread
250ml (10 fl oz) milk
half an onion, finely chopped
1 carrot, finely chopped
1 clove garlic, crushed
1 tablespoon (15ml) groundnut or sunflower oil
1–2 teaspoons (5–10ml) mild curry paste – use more if
   you have a curry fiend
150g (6 oz) free-flow frozen Vegemince
50g (2 oz) sultanas or ready-to-use dried apricots,
   chopped
1 tablespoon (15ml) mild mango chutney
1 banana, peeled and sliced lengthways
1 egg, beaten and made up to 125ml (5 fl oz) with
   milk

Pre-heat the oven to 180°C/350°F/Gas 4. Soak the bread in the milk. Fry the onion, carrot and garlic in the oil until starting to soften, add the curry paste and stir fry for a couple of minutes. Remove the bread from the milk and mix into the vegetable mixture. Add the milk used to soak the bread, the Vegemince, the sultanas or apricots and the mango chutney and stir well. Place this mixture in a greased oven-proof dish. Place the halved banana on top and pour over the egg and milk mixture. Bake in the pre-heated oven for 30–35 minutes until browning on top. Serve with rice.

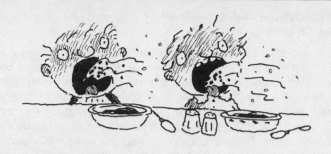

Cheese topped bean grill
Makes 1 meal

1 onion, chopped
1 tablespoon (15ml) groundnut or sunflower oil
100g (4 oz) button mushrooms, sliced
200g can chopped tomatoes
200g can butter beans, red kidney beans (drained) or
    baked beans in tomato sauce
few slices French bread or 1 slice white bread,
    buttered on one side
50g (2 oz) grated cheddar or gruyère cheese

Fry the onion in the oil for 5 minutes, then add the sliced
mushrooms and cook for a few minutes more to soften the
mushrooms. Add the tomatoes and your chosen beans (if
using baked beans add the sauce from the tin as well). Cook
gently for 5 minutes. Pre-heat the grill. Spoon the bean
mixture into a greased oven-proof dish and then place the
bread slices on top (if using a slice of white bread, cut into
triangles first). Sprinkle with the cheese and grill until the
cheese is bubbling and browning. Remove from the grill and
let the dish cool a little before serving as the cheese will still
be very hot. Melted cheese must be tested carefully before
giving to children as it retains its heat and children can easily
burn their mouths on it.

I sometimes also add some sliced tomatoes to this recipe,
putting them either under or on top of the cheese before
grilling. Serve with a fruit juice or a few sliced tomatoes if
you have not already added some.

Veggie sausage and apple loaf*
Makes 2 meals

I have made this recipe with a number of stuffing mixes, and feel that it is best not to go for ones that have too many herbs (particularly sage) in them, otherwise the finished loaf is very reminiscent of eating sage and onion stuffing! I use the frozen veggie sausages from the Linda McCartney range which are my children's favourites and hold their shape well. (I defrost them before chopping and cooking.) I also often substitute some of the boiling water with about 100ml (4 fl oz) of apple juice when making up the stuffing mix – this enhances the apple flavour.

113g pack of stuffing mix
300ml (12 fl oz) boiling water
1 leek, chopped
1 onion, chopped
3 veggie sausages, chopped
1 tablespoon (15ml) groundnut or sunflower oil
1 apple, peeled, cored and finely chopped

Pre-heat the oven to 180°C/350°F/Gas 4. Mix together the stuffing mix and water and leave to stand. Gently fry the leek, onion and sausages in the oil for 5 minutes until starting to soften. Mix into the stuffing mix with the chopped apple. Pack the mixture into a greased and lined 900g (2 lb) loaf tin. Bake in the pre-heated oven for 30–35 minutes until browning. Serve in slices or spoon out of the tin. Serve hot with vegetables and gravy or cold with salad and tomato ketchup or home-made tomato sauce (see page 155).

Tomato sauce
Makes 2–4 portions

1 onion, chopped
1 clove garlic, crushed (optional)
1 tablespoon (15ml) olive or sunflower oil
400g can chopped tomatoes

Fry the onion and garlic (if using) in the oil for 5–10 minutes until starting to brown (but not so that the onion is starting to blacken at the edges). Add the chopped tomatoes, cover and cook gently for 10 minutes. For very young or fussy eaters put the sauce through a mouli before using. Otherwise blend or use as it is.

Crunchy vegetable and tomato bake
Makes 1–2 meals

200g (8 oz) potato, diced
200g (8 oz) carrot, diced
100g (4 oz) swede or turnip, diced
50g (2 oz) butter
half a portion of tomato sauce (see above)
30g packet ready-salted crisps

Pre-heat the oven to 180°C/350°F/Gas 4. Place the potato, carrot and swede or turnip in a saucepan and cover with water. Bring to the boil and simmer for 15 minutes. Drain, return to the pan and roughly fork over. (This is how you make bashed neeps!) Add the butter and mix in. Spoon into a gratin dish and cover with the sauce. Bash the crisps lightly, just enough to break them up a little, not turn them into crumbs, and sprinkle them on top. Cook in the pre-heated oven for 20 minutes. Serve with broccoli or green beans.

Potato topped bean pie
Makes 1–2 meals

1 onion, chopped
1 carrot, chopped
1 tablespoon (15ml) groundnut or sunflower oil
150g (6 oz) mushrooms or courgettes, chopped
400g can chopped tomatoes
225g can red kidney beans or butter beans, drained, or
  baked beans in tomato sauce
400g (1 lb) mashed potato (made with butter and milk)
50g (2 oz) grated gruyère or cheddar cheese

Pre-heat the oven to 200°C/400°F/Gas 6. Fry the onion and carrot in the oil for 5 minutes and then add the mushrooms or courgettes and fry for a few minutes more until softening. Mix in the chopped tomatoes and whichever beans you are using. Spoon into a greased oven-proof dish and top with the mashed potato and then sprinkle with the grated cheese. Bake for 30 minutes until brown. Serve with fruit juice.

Savoury wedges*
Makes 3 meals

This is our most popular recipe using red lentils – although when first made its texture is very soft, on leaving it becomes firm enough to slice and take as a lunchbox or picnic food.

200g (8 oz) red split lentils
500ml (1 pint) water with 1 teaspoon (5ml) Marmite added
1 onion, chopped
knob of butter
150g (6 oz) grated gruyère or cheddar cheese
1 tablespoon (15ml) chopped fresh parsley
1 egg, beaten
3 tablespoons (approx 20 oz/50g) cooked rice
1 slice bread, crumbed
3 tablespoons (45ml) tomato ketchup or tomato sauce (see page 155)
30g packet ready-salted crisps, lightly broken up

Pre-heat the oven to 190°C/375°F/Gas 5. Cook the lentils in the Marmite and water until soft and until all the liquid has been absorbed – be careful not to burn. Meanwhile gently fry the onion in the butter until soft. When the lentils and onion are cooked, mix these with 100g (4 oz) of the grated cheese, the parsley, egg, rice and breadcrumbs. Mix well and pack into an oiled 20cm (8 in) cake tin (I use one with sprung sides which makes the finished dish easier to remove). Spread the tomato ketchup or sauce over the top and sprinkle with the remaining cheese and crisps. Bake in the pre-heated oven for 30 minutes. Cut into wedges and serve. Good hot or cold with broccoli and tomatoes.

Claire's ratatouille
Makes 1–2 meals

Our friend Claire passed this recipe on to me – it has been an enduring favourite with her son Brendan. It makes a great lunch dish served with crusty French bread and grated cheese or with pasta, rice or baked potatoes. Claire also uses it to make a vegetarian lasagne. When cooked for adults she often adds some red wine with the water. I hadn't come across a recipe for ratatouille that adds pearl barley but it works extremely well. This recipe shows how parents adjust recipes to suit their own offspring – most recipes would have more onion, but Brendan only likes a little onion and his penchant for raisins (as with many children) is well known, hence the unusual addition of raisins. You have to be adaptable when cooking for children!

> half an onion, chopped
> 1 medium aubergine, washed and chopped
> 3 medium courgettes, washed and chopped
> 2 tablespoons (30ml) olive oil
> 2 tablespoons (30ml) plain flour
> 2 tablespoons (30ml) tomato purée
> 200g can chopped tomatoes
> handful of pearl barley – about 2–3 tablespoons or 50g
>   (2 oz)
> handful of raisins – about 2–3 tablespoons or 50g
>   (2 oz)

Pre-heat the oven to 180°C/350°F/Gas 4. Fry the onion, aubergine and courgette in the oil for a few minutes, stir in the flour and then the tomato purée and tinned tomatoes. Keep stirring or will begin to stick (don't do this over a very high heat). Add enough water or wine to make a thick soup-like consistency. Add the pearl barley and raisins, and bring to the boil. If it now seems a little too thick add a touch more water or wine. Transfer to a casserole dish and cook in the pre-heated oven for 45 minutes.

Cheesy pasta and vegetable bake
Makes 2 meals

Although this is not Claire's recipe we have often had a similar dish when visiting Claire, and these pasta bakes tend to go down very well with most children.

150g (6 oz) penne or pasta bows
1 medium carrot, sliced
100g (4 oz) broccoli florets, sliced
4 tomatoes, each cut top to bottom into 6 segments
   (and skinned if cooking for a child under 1 year)
200g can sweetcorn, drained
500ml (1 pint) cheese sauce (see page 97)
50g (2 oz) fresh breadcrumbs
50g (2 oz) grated cheddar or gruyère cheese

Pre-heat the oven to 200°C/400°F/Gas 6. Cook the pasta as directed on the packet. Meanwhile place the carrots in a saucepan and cover with water, bring to the boil and simmer for 4 minutes before placing a steamer on top and steaming the broccoli in this for another 4 minutes. Drain the cooked pasta and vegetables and mix these with the tomatoes, sweetcorn and cheese sauce. Place in a greased oven-proof dish. Mix together the breadcrumbs and grated cheese and use this mixture to top the bake. Place in the pre-heated oven and cook for 25 minutes until brown on top. Serve with a fruit juice.

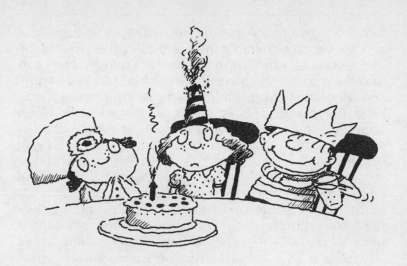

8. Party time

Toddlers love parties! We managed to get away with not having a party when James was one but not when Helena turned one as by then James had caught on that birthdays mean parties. (He was two and three-quarters). So although Helena was oblivious to the fact that she was having a birthday, James would have been very upset if we hadn't had a party for her. As father unfortunately was away in Australia that week this was quite a feat for mother to arrange. However, it was done and Helena had a really lovely time.

The two really important features of toddlers' parties are the birthday cake (with candles) and balloons – if these are present you can really get away with a simple tea and, when very little, just one or two games. To be honest I think that the simpler you keep the party the better it will be as in these tender years their expectations are not too high.

When they are very young you can also cheerfully

mix the ages of their guests, but when they reach four and are very much into games and rules then to mix the age groups can be disastrous as the younger ones can 'spoil' the game for the older ones. You can only really consider having your child's party in your home if you have the space. This is easier in the summer when hopefully you will have access to the garden, but what will your contingency plan be if it does pour with rain on the day? I think that this is why so many other venues for children's parties have sprung up – and of course the fact that you won't have to clear up your home (and possible accidents) after the event. Incidentally, something else to think about when planning a party at home – if you have family pets, think about where you will put them when the guests arrive because boisterous children and pets do not mix well.

So here are some of the best party themes that we have come across, and hopefully some new ideas for parties and party food.

Tiny tots

For the ones and twos stick to a very simple tea party or picnic. The only decorations that you will need are balloons – but make sure that you have enough for all the guests to be able to take one home and that your children will still have some left, or there will be tears and tantrums. A simple sponge cake will do for the birthday cake – it doesn't even have to be iced – but you will need one or two birthday candles because even if your little one wouldn't miss these the older guests will. You can of course buy a birthday cake – all the supermarkets have them. It is possible just to pick one up on the day but if you want a particular design you should order it or pick it up a few days in advance to make sure that you get the one that you want. Try

162

and keep the numbers down, as there will be a lot of children just running around and letting off steam, and make sure just a few toys are around for the guests to play with – ones without lots of parts are best or the mess will be terrible. We tried playing 'the farmer's in his den' but it wasn't very successful. At this age their concentration span is very limited and your chances of getting all of your guests' attention at the same time are fairly limited. We did find that 'pass the parcel' went down very well – with a tiny gift in each layer of wrapping (little packets of chocolate buttons, balloons, farm animals and crayons were all well received). Make sure that the person controlling the music can see what's happening so that you can rig the game to ensure that the gifts are fairly evenly distributed. The music can be a child's tape – there are many with songs and rhymes on them which are suitable for children's parties – or a tape or CD of your own with some 'upbeat' music on it. Most children do like dancing and will often start of their own accord if the music appeals to them.

At this age the main event is going to be the birthday tea so don't have more then half an hour between the guests arriving and tea. I would suggest that a half-past three start is suitable, with tea at four o'clock, then the guests will be ready to leave by five o'clock. You can buy tableware at supermarkets and specialist party shops and some large toy shops or warehouses sell it as well.

At Helena's party I decorated the table by placing sweets (such as Smarties, Liquorice Allsorts and chocolate buttons) all around the place settings – this proved to be a very popular idea with the children. I also tied a helium balloon to each chair or highchair and this helped to keep the very young ones amused. Don't go overboard on the food – think how much your children eat at tea and multiply this by the number of guests, adding just a little in case some have bigger appetites than your little darlings. A guide for this age group is one or two bite-sized sandwiches, one or two savouries, one or two sweet items or jelly and ice-cream or creamy topping.

It is perfectly possible to buy in all the party food; it may not be the healthiest option but in some cases if the party is going to come off at all then you may not have the time to prepare much food. As Andy was away when Helena's birthday came round I found that I had no time at all to prepare any food, and as it was a snap decision to have the party I had not had any time to cook ahead and put food in the freezer as I had done at Christmas. It was very easy to buy food in from supermarkets and then all I had to do on the day was make a few sandwiches and using canapé cutters make them the right size for the little ones. I even found some cartons of yoghurt and jelly in the chilled cabinets. So don't feel guilty if you have to resort to buying in items, the party will be more enjoyable if the parent is not frazzled from having prepared it.

Most children learn very quickly to expect a little party bag at the end of a party. I have to admit that a lot of what goes into these bags can easily be a waste of money. For this age group it is difficult to decide on goodies to take away as many will still be putting items in their mouths. For Helena's party I decided on sweets and chocolates (which are definitely approved of by the children) and to appease the mums I added a toothbrush! I matched the children's age to appropriate sweets and made a little bag from the napkins, which, tied with ribbon, made a lovely little party bag to take home.

Tiny tots' party checklist

- Invitations (or you can just phone)

- Order or make cake – don't forget to buy the candles and candle holders (do you have matches?)

- Buy or order balloons, ribbon, tableware, party prizes or gifts, bags, presents

- Wrap up parcel/s for pass the parcel

- Ensure you have some suitable music

- Decide on food – make up shopping list

- Food shop

- Prepare food

- Clear party room

- Decorate house, room and table

- Pick up cake, balloons if necessary

- Make up party bags

- Put out a few toys for guests

- Finally make sure that you have decided in advance what you and your child or children will be wearing and that everything is clean and ready to wear, otherwise the chances are that it will be in the wash or waiting to be ironed!

Suggested party food

Bite-sized sandwiches, tiny sausages or sausage rolls, fingers or little wedges of pizza, assorted crisps or nibbles, shaped biscuits, tiny muffins or cupcakes or jelly with ice-cream or creamy topping and, of course, a birthday cake.

Toddlers' teddy bear picnic

For James' second birthday we had a picnic (indoors as it turned out). This was very easy to organise and I can strongly recommend it, especially if the birthday falls in the summer and you have a reasonable chance of fine weather. We also used this idea of a teddy bears' picnic at James' christening as it did take place in fine weather and we were able to use the garden – it kept the little ones amused for ages, in fact one young man just sat there quietly chomping away for most of the afternoon!

Limit the party to two hours; this will allow plenty of time for tea and a couple of games or dancing and just generally letting off steam. Even if you are having your picnic outdoors keep the numbers in check – five to eight little friends should suffice, especially if mums are having to bring baby brothers or sisters. Again for this age group you can still quite happily mix the children's ages and we didn't attempt any organised games. If the weather is fine most children will play quite happily in the garden without too much intervention – just the parents' presence is needed. However, indoors you may want to have a couple of games to play and you will need a music tape. Again use either a children's party tape or a tape or CD of your own.

We actually just used our children's bears for the picnic but you could make a point of asking the guests to bring a teddy of their own, making out the invitations to the child and his teddy. There are lots of invites that feature teddies (I've seen some really lovely ones with Winnie-the-Pooh on them). Or you can make your own either making a teddy-shaped card or cutting out a teddy from some coloured card and sticking this onto a piece of card. You could then dress the teddy with a ribbon necktie and coloured party hat, or have him holding a party balloon. Don't forget when making invitations to choose your envelopes first then make the card to fit the envelope. At this age I think the invitation is very important and especially that it should come through the post, which is a real treat for the child.

For a picnic the one essential is a couple of picnic rugs so look yours out or buy some paper tablecloths that will act as picnic rugs. With this age group you don't really need plates as they will just pick from the platters of food. I put two platters out with the same selection of food on each so no child should have too far to reach to get at the food. At this age the cake is starting to be important to the birthday child so if buying one try and get one with a teddy theme. A cake with a teddy outline on it is very easy to do, one made in a teddy shape is more difficult but not impossible – and I'm certainly no expert at cake decoration. At this age children still have very small appetites so there is no need to allow any more food than you would do for a tiny tots' party – one or two bite-sized sandwiches, one or two savouries, one or two sweet items.

For the party bags I picked one small toy or plastic mug suitable for each child's age, some sweets or chocolates, a balloon and a little book or colouring leaflet – don't forget to mark who the recipient of the bag will be. And when the children are leaving don't forget to remind them to take their bears home as well!

Toddlers' teddy bear picnic checklist

- Invitations

- Organise the cake and candles, etc.

- Search out picnic rugs or put paper tablecloths on your shopping list

- Decide if you are having any party games and organise these (with prizes if necessary)

- Buy or order the balloons, ribbon, platters for food, party bags, prizes or gifts

- Decide on suitable music (if outside will you need batteries for your tape machine?)

- Decide on food

- Food shop

- Prepare food

- Clear up garden or party room

- Pick up cake, balloons if necessary

- Make up party bags

- Put out a few toys for when the guests arrive

- Make sure you and your child or children are spick and span before the guests arrive

Suggested party food

Bite-sized sandwiches, crudités and dips, chicken nuggets, assorted crisps and nibbles, Smartie cakes, chocolate squares or crispies (or ice-cream lollies) and the birthday cake.

Thrilling threes party

At this age children will be thrilled to dress up for the party, but choose an easy theme for the poor parents who have to make up the costume. I think it is a good idea to give the parents some ideas so the two themes that I have chosen are 'rhymes and fairy tales' and 'a scarecrow party'.

Rhymes and fairy tales

This is a very easy one as the characters are so diverse the children can come as almost anyone or anything, and parents can get plenty of ideas on how to dress their children just by looking at books of rhymes or fairy tales. Witches, fairies and characters such as Little Red Riding Hood or Alice in Wonderland will appeal to little girls. Animals, giants, soldiers, farmers and kings will appeal to little boys.

At this age they are very keen on rhymes and will happily spend some time performing these – favourites are 'Ring-a-ring-a-roses', 'The grand old Duke of York' and 'The wheels on the bus go round and round'.

A scarecrow party

This again is easy to achieve, the main essential being some straw or hay (which can be bought cheaply at any pet shop). Then the child can dress as messily as possible with bits of straw sticking out from pockets, cuffs, under a hat, etc. If you have some very old clothes that are about to be thrown out you can use these very effectively by making a hole at a knee or elbow and arranging some straw so that it looks as if some of the scarecrow's stuffing is coming out. You could of course expand this theme to include farmyard animals, farmers, milkmaids, etc.

Suitable rhymes for the children to perform would be 'Dingle-dangle scarecrow', 'Old MacDonald' and 'The farmer's in his den'.

Organising a thrilling threes party

I would still limit the party to two hours as parents still have to accompany their children and may have other offspring with them.

Find suitable invitations or make themed invitations of your own. You could photocopy some pictures of characters and stick them on a card or cut out a scarecrow from coloured card and stick this on a piece of card, adding yellow wool for the hair and a piece of stuffing escaping from his knee.

I would buy a plain tablecloth for these themes and stick cut-out characters onto this. Find appropriate tableware and when decorating the party room use balloons and party streamers. If having a scarecrow party outside as a picnic, splash out on a couple of bales of hay and checked tablecloths to add character.

You can buy a cake – chocolate caterpillar cakes are very popular with this age group or make a gingerbread house or scarecrow cake. Party blowers are popular with this age group as are balloon squeals, both of which can be bought at party shops (and added to the party bags at the end). Other goodies for the bags could include a cheap book of rhymes or a fairy tale or a book with farm animals featured; small colouring books or crayons are also good gift ideas. Another welcome gift is a small farm animal.

Thrilling threes party checklist

- Invitations

- Buy or order the cake, including candles, etc.

- Decide on games and organise these (with prizes if necessary)

- Buy or order balloons, ribbon, decorations (hay bales, etc.), tableware, party bags, gifts or prizes

- Organise suitable music

- Decide on party food

- Food shop

- Prepare food

- Clear out party room or garden

- Decorate the party room or arrange garden for party

- Pick up cake, balloons (if necessary)

- Make up party bags

- Make sure that your child's or children's party costume is ready.

Suggested party food

Sandwiches made with animal cutters, sandwich snails, pizza faces, novelty chicken pieces, assorted crisps and snacks, mice cakes, gingerbread shapes, the birthday cake.

Fearsome fours

At this age some of your child's friends may already have started at school, so the party will either have to be at the weekend or start after school has finished (and allowing the children time to get home and get changed). Again a themed party will go down well but choose a more active theme. The two examples that I have chosen are pirates and a space party.

Costumes are easily made with eye patches and scarves tied around their heads and waists (and possibly moustaches painted on their faces) for the pirates and the judicious use of cardboard boxes (either with or without silver spray). Look at Andy in *Toy Story* to see how easily a cardboard box can turn you into a spaceman. Silver foil can also be used to cut out stars and planets and these stuck onto a long drawstring skirt if girls want a more glamorous outfit. Silver tinsel can be wrapped around the head or face paint used to make glamorous or weird aliens.

Invitations can be made featuring the skull and crossbones or in the shape of a spaceship. Paper chains are good decorations (use metallic ones for a space party) and your children will enjoy making them up.

Games will definitely need to be organised for this age group (and you will find that they are very strict about rules for these). Musical chairs, statues or bumps are all very popular with this age group. The 'space-man's walk' or 'pirate's jig' can be played as well – while the music plays the spacemen must walk very slowly, arms out and only one foot on the ground at a time, while the pirates must cross their arms and hop up and down on one leg. When the music stops they must keep absolutely still – anyone who wobbles is out. Those who are out can help you spot the wobblers. The last one in is the winner.

Another good game is the 'black spot' or 'spaceman's madness'. For this you will need one small circle of black card for each child playing the game. The mums stand in one line and the children in another. The child at the start of the line puts their black spot in one hand and then steps forward with hands clenched and the first mother has to choose one of the child's hands. When the child opens that hand, if the black spot is revealed the child has to go to the back of the line of children; if the black spot was in the other hand the child moves on to the next mother and the game is repeated. The next child comes forward to the first mother and tries their luck. To win the child has to get through the line of mothers. (If more than five children are playing this game it is better to have two lines.)

Most children also love 'ladybird, ladybird fly away home'. For the spacemen, get them to face you and make sure each child has plenty of room. Explain that you will call out the names of different birds and animals, some of which can fly. If they think that the bird or animal that you have named can fly, they must flap their arms, but keep them down by their sides if it cannot. If they get it wrong they are out and must watch the others and tell you if they get it wrong. Call out the names slowly at first and then faster and faster to try and confuse them. For the pirates play the game with animals or fish that swim and get them to do swimming motions with their arms.

Probably the most well-received game is a treasure hunt. You will need plenty of little prizes, wrapped and hidden around the party room or garden (wrap them in pirate flags or silver foil). The children all have to search for the hidden 'treasure'. You can make this game last a little longer by playing music and only letting them search for the treasure while the music is stopped. This leads to much excitement, so be prepared to play a quiet game afterwards (such as pass the parcel) to calm them down again.

Party bags can include fake noses and moustaches,

bubble blowers, whistles or key rings, or novelty pencil sharpeners or erasers.

Fearsome fours party checklist

- Invitations

- Order or make the cake

- Decide on games and organise (with prizes if necessary)

- Buy or order balloons, ribbon, tableware, decorations, party bags, prizes, gifts

- Organise suitable music

- Decide on party food

- Food shop

- Prepare food

- Clear out party room

- Decorate party room

- Pick up cake, balloons (if necessary)

- Make up party bags

- Ensure your child's/children's costume is ready.

Suggested party food

Small sandwiches made using star or fish cutters, sausage whirlpools, celery boats, pizza faces or planets, chicken nuggets, filo stars or parcels, chocolate nuggets, and for the birthday cake either buy one that will fit the theme or make a pirate or spaceship cake. At this age I would allow about two to three sandwiches, three to four savouries and two to three sweet items.

You don't, of course, have to hold your child's birthday party at home. There are now many venues that can be hired, some of which will cater for the children as well. Possible venues are fast-food restaurants; swimming pools; local halls – if you seek out one used by a mother and toddler group, you may well be also able to hire small tables and chairs with a collection of toys for your little guests; farms and zoos; or most attractions aimed at families with small children.

You can also hire other attractions such as bouncy castles – I found a very comprehensive list of children's facilities at our local library. Children's entertainers can also be hired, but do ensure that they will be suitable for your guests – when children are very little, some may find these entertainers too frightening. At two and a half, James wept copiously at the sight of a magic entertainer twisting balloons into animals and making things appear and disappear.

Recipes for children's parties

I have included recipes for the parties above and also a few bits and pieces that can be made and stuck in the freezer – useful in the picnic season and in the rush up to Christmas when most children will have many parties to attend and mothers need to send a food contribution.

Sandwiches

Don't go overboard on these as most children will eat only one or two. Make them with a mixture of brown and white bread – choose thin- or medium-cut loaves. You can try a speciality bread – I have found walnut bread to be popular with many children but cut it very thinly. Fillings that many children will eat include: grated cheese, Dairylea and Marmite, cucumber and Marmite, peanut butter, and thinly cut ham. Sandwich together the slices of bread with your chosen filling, then remove crusts and cut into either four or eight sandwiches. If you have some canapé cutters, you could do as I did at Helena's party and cut the different fillings with differing canapé cutters. Heart-, diamond- and star-shaped sandwiches are very appealing. You can also make pinwheels by just spreading one slice of crustless bread with your filling and then rolling it up (like a Swiss roll) and cutting it into circular slices.

Sandwich snails
Makes 12

> 100g (4 oz) cream cheese
> 1 tablespoon (15ml) mayonnaise
> 4 slices crustless bread
> 12 small cherry tomatoes

Mix together the cream cheese and mayonnaise and spread this over the slices of bread. Roll up as for a swiss roll but leave about a quarter to a third of the bread unrolled. Cut each roll into 3 slices and place a small cherry tomato on the unrolled part of the bread for the snail's 'head'.

Savouries

Tiny sausages that have already been cooked can be bought at most large supermarkets (they usually come in packs of 50) and sausage rolls can be bought frozen in large rolls which you then cut to your required size.

Chicken nuggets in all shapes and sizes can be found in both the freezer and chilled cabinets in supermarkets. I'm not a great fan of these, but they are invariably popular with children (I have found that the chilled ones are better). You can also buy vegetarian versions of these products.

Crudités and dips can also be bought ready made from supermarkets but here is a selection we have made that has been popular with small guests. Serve these dips with fingers of fresh courgette, carrot, cucumber or pepper, little florets of cauliflower and cherry tomatoes for dipping.

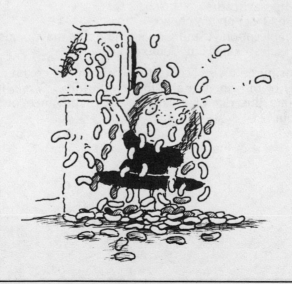

Creamy cheese dip
Makes 6–8 portions

> 100g (4 oz) cream cheese
> 2 tablespoons (30ml) Greek yoghurt
> pinch of fresh chopped chives (optional)

Cream together the cheese and yoghurt until you have a blended creamy dip, add the chives if using and serve.

Peanut butter dip
Makes 6–8 portions

> 100g (4 oz) smooth peanut butter
> 4 tablespoons (60ml) Greek yoghurt
> about half a teaspoon of Marmite

Cream together the smooth peanut butter and the yoghurt until well blended. Add just a taste of Marmite and beat this in. Serve.

Avocado and cheese dip
Makes 6–8 portions

> 1 ripe avocado
> 75g (3 oz) cream cheese
> 1 tablespoon (15ml) Greek yoghurt or mayonnaise
> 1 tablespoon (15ml) lemon juice

Mash or purée the avocado, then beat in the cream cheese, yoghurt or mayonnaise and the lemon juice. Serve. Do not refrigerate this dip or make too far in advance or it will discolour.

Tomato straws
Makes 40

    50g (2 oz) plain flour
    25g (1 oz) margarine
    25g (1 oz) grated cheddar or parmesan cheese
    1 medium egg yolk, beaten
    1 tablespoon (15ml) tomato purée

Pre-heat the oven to 200°C/400°F/Gas 6. Using your finger-tips rub together the flour and margarine until you have a mixture that resembles breadcrumbs. Mix in the grated cheese. Add the other ingredients and mix to a firm dough (you can do all this very quickly in a food processor). On a lightly floured surface, roll out the dough thinly into a rectangle about 12 × 18cm (5 × 7 inches). Cut in half and then cut each rectangle into thin strips (about 5mm or ¼ inch each). This should make about 20 strips from each rectangle. Give each strip a slight twist as you place it on a baking sheet and bake for about 8 minutes in the pre-heated oven until golden. Cool on a wire rack.

Cheese bites
Makes 37

Just before Christmas I bought a hexagonal canapé cutter from Lakeland Plastics and I have been very impressed with the resulting little pastry parcels that I have made using it. I made lots of little mince pies with it which were just right for children's parties, but here I give my recipe for little pies with a cheese filling. You could make these by lining little canapé tins with the pastry, filling them and topping with more pastry.

Cheese pastry
175g (7 oz) plain flour
pinch mustard powder
75g (3 oz) margarine
50g (2 oz) finely grated cheddar cheese
1 egg yolk

Cheese filling
150g (6 oz) cream cheese
50g (2 oz) finely grated cheddar cheese
little milk or beaten egg for glazing

Either rub the flour, mustard powder and margarine together to produce a crumb mixture, or whizz together in a food processor. Stir in the cheese and then blend in the egg yolk. This should form a dough. Add a little cold water if more moisture is needed to form a soft dough. Dust the canapé cutter with flour and then roll out half of the dough into a large circle which will cover the cutter. Mix together the filling and divide among the canapés. Roll out the rest of the dough and use this to cover the filling. Use your rolling pin to separate the canapés and then knock them out onto a baking sheet. Chill for 15 minutes. Pre-heat the oven to 200°C/400°F/Gas 6. Brush the canapés with a little milk or beaten egg before baking in the pre-heated oven for 10 minutes or until golden brown.

Pizza shapes
Makes 24–30

A multitude of pizzas can be bought and then cooked and cut into small fingers or wedges. However, here are a few home-made ones that you may like to try and that really don't take very long to make.

> 1 packet pizza base mix
> 2 tablespoons (30ml) tomato purée
> 2 tablespoons (30ml) tomato ketchup
> 200g (8 oz) grated cheddar or mozzarella cheese (you can buy bags of ready grated cheeses for pizza in supermarkets)

Pre-heat the oven to 200°C/400°F/Gas 6. Make up the pizza dough as directed on the packet. Roll out on a floured surface, as thinly as you can. Using small biscuit cutters, cut the dough into little shapes (the number you will have depends on how thinly you have rolled the dough out and the size of your cutters). Re-roll the leftover dough to get as many shapes as possible. Mix together the tomato purée and tomato ketchup and spread a little of this mixture on each shape. Sprinkle with the cheese and then place on baking sheets. Cook in the pre-heated oven for 8–14 minutes (smaller shapes will cook more quickly). Can be served warm or cold.

Pizza fingers
Makes 24

1 packet pizza base mix
3 tablespoons (45ml) tomato purée
2 tablespoons (30ml) tomato ketchup
200g (8 oz) grated cheddar or mozzarella cheese, or a
  mixture of both

Pre-heat the oven to 200°C/400°F/Gas 6. Make up the pizza dough as directed on the packet. Roll out on a floured surface to fit into the bottom of an 18 × 28cm (7 × 11 inches) baking tray. Press in evenly, making sure that it goes right up to the edges and into the corners. Prick all over the dough with a fork. Mix together the tomato purée and tomato ketchup and spread this all over the dough. Sprinkle with the grated cheeses. Bake in the pre-heated oven for 12–15 minutes until cheese is melting and browning. Leave in the tin for a few minutes and then remove to a wire rack to cool. Trim the edges and cut into 24 fingers before serving.

These pizza recipes are very simple, and I have found the simple ones to be the most popular with very young children. As the children get a little older you could start getting more adventurous and adding herbs and other toppings such as sliced meats and vegetables, sweetcorn, pineapple pieces, etc.

Pizza faces, planets, etc.
Makes 10–12 portions

1 pizza dough base
3 tablespoons (45ml) tomato purée
2 tablespoons (30ml) tomato ketchup
75g (3 oz) grated cheddar cheese
couple of slices of red Leicester cheese
a few chives
some red pepper
a courgette
some frozen peas

Pre-heat the oven to 200°C/400°F/Gas 6. Make up the pizza dough as directed on the packet. Cut out some circles about 10cm (3–4 inches) in diameter. Mix together the tomato purée and the tomato ketchup and spread over the pizza circles. Now decorate your pizzas – plainer garnishes tend to look better than overdoing it. Use the other ingredients to make the pizzas into faces or planets. The red Leicester cheese can be cut into triangles for use as ears for animals or grated and used to make planets of different hues, or hair for faces. The red pepper can be used to make rings for planets, or noses or mouths for faces. Thinly cut chives can be used as animal whiskers for faces. Peas are good for eyes and the courgette can be thinly sliced into shapes for eyes, noses or mouths for faces. Bake in the pre-heated oven for 10–12 minutes.

Sausage whirlpools
Makes 12–16

> 250g (10 oz) puff pastry
> 250g (10 oz) pork and apricot or pork and apple
> sausagemeat
> 1 egg, beaten

Pre-heat the oven to 200°C/400°F/Gas 6. Roll out the pastry into a rectangle about 18 × 28cm (7 × 11 inches). Spread with the sausagemeat then roll up like a Swiss roll. Cut into thin circles and place on a baking tray. Brush with the beaten egg and bake in the pre-heated oven for 15–20 minutes until golden brown. Cool before serving.

Celery boats
Makes 12

> 3 celery sticks
> 100g (4 oz) cream cheese
> 50g (2 oz) cooked shredded chicken or ham
> 3 cheese slices
> 12 triangular-shaped corn chips

Start by cutting each celery stick into four small lengths that can be used as the base of the boats. Slice a tiny slither off the bottom of each so that it sits upright. Mix the cream cheese with the cooked meat and use this to stuff the boats. Now cut the cheese slices into triangles for a sail for each boat, stick these at the front of each boat and then insert a corn chip next to it as the second sail.

Sweet things

Biscuit shapes
Makes 20–30

Make these biscuits a couple of days in advance but don't decorate until the day – leave some time for the icing to harden before serving. These are the sort of biscuits that your children will love to help you to make – they will eat the dough too if you don't watch them!

> 150g (6 oz) plain flour, sifted
> half a teaspoon (2.5ml) ground cinnamon
> pinch ground ginger
> 75g (3 oz) unsalted butter
> 25g (1 oz) caster sugar
> 50g (2 oz) runny honey
> tubes of icing for decorating

Mix together the sifted flour, the cinnamon and the ginger. Cream together the butter and sugar and then add the honey, blend well and gradually add the flour and spice mixture, beating well. Wrap the dough in cling film and refrigerate for a few hours. When you are ready to bake your biscuits, pre-heat the oven to 180°C/350°F/Gas 4. Line a baking sheet/s with greaseproof paper or baking parchment and roll out the dough thinly. Using biscuit cutters, cut into biscuit shapes and place on the baking sheets. Bake for about 10 minutes until a light brown in colour. Leave to cool and then decorate with the icing.

Chocolate mini muffins
Makes 12

Muffins are incredibly easy to make as long as you follow one rule – do not overmix.

> 1 medium egg, beaten
> 4 tablespoons (60ml) milk
> 25g (1 oz) butter, melted
> 75g (3 oz) plain flour
> 1 tablespoon (15ml) cocoa powder
> 1 teaspoon (5ml) baking powder
> 25g (1 oz) caster sugar
> 50g (2 oz) chocolate buttons (roughly broken)

Pre-heat the oven to 200°C/400°F/Gas 6. Lightly mix together the egg, milk and melted butter. Sieve in the flour, cocoa powder and baking powder, add the sugar and chocolate buttons and very lightly and quickly fold together. Do not overmix. Divide the mixture between 12 mini muffin cases and bake in the pre-heated oven for 10 minutes until risen. Transfer to a cooling tray (in their cases).

Chocolate squares
Makes 24

> 200g (8 oz) plain cooking chocolate
> 75g (3 oz) margarine or butter
> 3 tablespoons (45ml) runny honey
> 300g (12 oz) digestive biscuits, crushed
> 24 Maltesers

Melt the chocolate, margarine or butter and honey. Stir in the crushed biscuits and mix thoroughly. Turn into a greased and lined 18 × 28cm (7 × 11 inches) baking tin. Spacing the Maltesers equally apart, and making 4 lines of 6 Maltesers, push them down into the mixture. Leave to set and then cut into squares with a Malteser in the middle of each square.

Cupcakes
Makes about 16

100g (4 oz) margarine or butter
100g (4 oz) caster sugar
100g (4 oz) self-raising flour
1 teaspoon (5ml) baking powder
2 eggs, beaten

Pre-heat the oven to 190°C/375°F/Gas 5. Cream together the margarine or butter and sugar and then beat in the flour, baking powder and eggs. Spread 16 paper cases over a baking sheet and divide the mixture between them. Bake in the pre-heated oven for 15–20 minutes until golden brown. Cool on a wire rack.

These can be made into Smartie cakes by decorating with a little icing and pressing a Smartie into the icing, or into lemon cakes by adding a little lemon zest and a teaspoonful of lemon juice to the mixture. Alternatively make into fairy cakes by cutting a slice off the top of the cake and then adding some buttercream to the top, cutting the cake slice in half and placing the 'wings' on top of the buttercream. Mice cakes can be made by topping the cakes with some white icing, using some red icing to draw on a nose and some ears and then using chocolate icing to draw on two eyes and some whiskers.

Chocolate nuggets (crispies)
Makes 16–20

150g (6 oz) plain cooking chocolate
25g (1 oz) raisins
100g (4 oz) puffed rice crispies

Break the chocolate up and place in a glass bowl, gently melt it over some boiling water or in the microwave. Mix with the raisins and crispies and divide among some paper cases. Leave to set.

Gingerbread shapes
Makes 12

25g (1 oz) margarine
50g (2 oz) soft dark brown sugar
2 tablespoons (30ml) golden syrup
100g (4 oz) plain flour
1 teaspoon (5ml) ground ginger
pinch of ground cinnamon
1 teaspoon (5ml) milk
half a teaspoon (2.5ml) bicarbonate of soda

Pre-heat the oven to 170°C/325°F/Gas 3. Melt the margarine, sugar and syrup, then mix with the other ingredients to form a soft dough. Put in a plastic bag and chill for 30 minutes. Roll out on a floured surface and use gingerbread cutters to cut out your gingerbread shapes. Place on a greased baking sheet. Bake in the pre-heated oven for 10–15 minutes, or until firm to the touch. Place on a wire rack to cool. If you wish you can decorate them with icing.

Filo stars or parcels
Makes 12

1 packet filo pastry, defrosted
12 dessertspoons (120ml) mincemeat
melted butter

Pre-heat the oven to 190°C/375°F/Gas 5. Cut the filo pastry into 36 squares. Using a 12-hole bun tin, put 3 filo squares in each hole, layering them at a slight angle so that each consists of a 12-pointed 'star'. Now put 1 dessertspoon of mincemeat into each star. Either scrunch each point up slightly to form a 'star' case or gather each star point up and scrunch together to form a 'parcel'. Then brush your star or parcel with melted butter. Now bake for about 10 minutes until crisp and brown.

Fruit jellies with creamy topping
Makes 4–6 depending on the size of your dishes

> 1 sachet sugar-free jelly crystals (to make 500ml or 1
>   pint of jelly)
> 33g sachet sugar-free Dream Topping mix
> 150ml (6 fl oz) milk

Measure 250ml (10 fl oz) boiling water into a jug, sprinkle
on the jelly crystals and stir to dissolve. Top up to the 500ml
(1 pint) mark with cold water. Divide between your dishes
and refrigerate. When set, put the milk in a bowl and
sprinkle on the Dream Topping mix, whisk for 2–3 minutes
until light and fluffy. Spread over the jellies and refrigerate
until needed. These can be made a day in advance and
stored in the refrigerator.

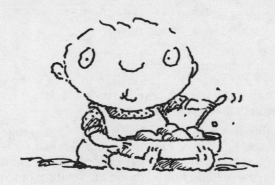

Cakes

It is essential that you have the right size of cake tins for your cake, so I have given recipes for both 18 and 20cm (7 and 8 inch) deep-sided sandwich cake tins. If you try and use cake tins that are too small, when the cake mixture rises it will come over the edges and form a hard crust on top which will spoil the result and make it very difficult to get out of the tin.

Basic birthday cake recipe
Makes 1 × 18cm cake (7 inch)

150g (6 oz) margarine or butter
150g (6 oz) caster sugar
3 eggs, beaten
150g (6 oz) self-raising flour, sifted
1 teaspoon (5ml) baking powder

To decorate
jam or buttercream (or both)
icing sugar or ready-made icing, fondant icing or
    frosting (all can be bought ready made)
chosen decorations, candles, trimmings

Pre-heat the oven to 180°C/350°F/Gas 4. Cream together the fat and sugar. Gradually beat in the eggs (add a little flour at this stage to ensure that the eggs do not curdle). Finally fold in the rest of the sifted flour. Divide the mixture between two greased and lined 18cm (7 inch) sandwich tins. Bake in the pre-heated oven for 20–25 minutes, or until they are well risen, brown and 'springy' to the touch, and starting to shrink slightly from the edges of the tins. Turn out onto a wire rack to cool. Sandwich together with your chosen filling/s and decorate in your chosen style.

Chocolate cake
Makes 1 × 20cm (8 inch) cake

200g (8 oz) self-raising flour
2 teaspoons (10ml) baking powder
2 tablespoons (30ml) cocoa powder mixed with 3
    tablespoons (45ml) boiling water
200g (8 oz) caster sugar
200g (8 oz) soft margarine
4 eggs

Pre-heat the oven to 180°C/350°F/Gas 4. Place all the
ingredients in a large bowl and mix well. Spoon into two
greased and lined 20cm (8 inch) cake tins. Bake in the
pre-heated oven for 25 minutes or until risen and brown.
Turn out onto a wire rack. When cool, sandwich together
with a chosen filling.

Buttercream
Enough for 18 fairy cakes or to fill and top one 8-inch cake

150g (6 oz) butter, softened
300g (12 oz) icing sugar, sifted

Cream together the butter and sugar until you have a smooth
cream. You can use this either by itself or with a layer of jam
to sandwich together cakes. To make chocolate buttercream,
to the above amounts add 2 tablespoons (30ml) cocoa
powder and 3 tablespoons (45ml) hot water. To make coffee
(mocha) buttercream add 2 tablespoons (30ml) coffee
essence.

Frosting
Enough to top one 8-inch cake or a traybake

Americans use 'frosting' on their cakes. It is usually spread over the cake and then a knife is used to pull it up into little peaks. A true frosting needs a sugar thermometer – but here is a recipe that I learnt when still at school!

    1 medium egg white
    175g (7 oz) caster sugar
    2 tablespoons (30ml) hot water
    pinch of cream of tartar

Put all of the ingredients into a glass bowl and whisk lightly. Place the bowl over a pan of simmering water and continue to whisk until the mixture has become so thick it will hold 'peaks' – this will take 7–10 minutes. You must use the frosting immediately, as it begins to set.

Decorating cakes

If, like me, you really are not very good at decorating cakes then one simple way is to make a round cake and then make a stencil of your chosen theme – say a teddy bear shape or a spaceship. Use this to either coat the cake with icing sugar or cocoa powder or use the stencil to trace the outline using ready-made icing tubes. However, there are a couple of designs I have not found too difficult to accomplish. But be warned that whenever you start to make cakes that stray from being just a plain shape you do incur a lot of wastage.

Teddy cake

As well as your 18cm (7 inch) cake you will need a smaller cake of about 7cm (3 inches). You will also need three Swiss rolls and a lot of icing (glacé or fondant) or frosting.

Lie your 18cm (7 inch) cake on a large cake board (this is the body) and then take a little semi circle out of the smaller cake so that it will sit at the top of the body (this is the head). For the ears take a slice from each of two of the Swiss rolls and sit these on the head as you have sat the head on the body. Using the two Swiss rolls that you have cut slices from, place these at the bottom of the body to act as the legs. Halve the last Swiss roll and use as the arms. Cover with icing and when set add eyes and mouth. A ribbon around the 'neck' looks good as well.

Gingerbread house cake

Make a rectangular cake (using the recipe for iced lemon cake on page 211 or coffee and pecan bake on page 212), ice or cover with frosting, and use Smarties and other sweets to mark out the roof tiles, door and windows. (Look in a fairy tale book for an illustration to help you.)

Scarecrow cake
Use a round cake and draw on a face with icing. Use liquorice strands for the hair.

Pirate cake
Use a rectangular cake and decorate with the skull and crossbones.

Spaceship cake
Either use a round cake and using a stencil draw on a spaceship or use a rectangular cake cut in half – one rectangle is the body of the spaceship and from the other rectangle cut out the nose and boosters. Cover with icing.

Although I have given you some ideas as to how you may decorate your birthday cake, you are of course only limited by your imagination. And although, like me, you may not be particularly good at decorating cakes at this stage, just imagine how good we could be by the time they are eighteen!

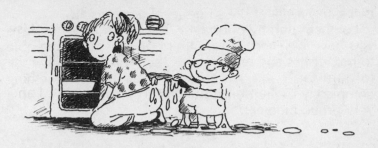

9. Baking and desserts

Although we should not be encouraging our children to get into the habit of eating lots of fatty and sugary dishes, it is perfectly okay for them to eat these foods occasionally. After all, we all like our treats. It is also good for the children to get into the kitchen and help with some cooking, and baking is a good area to get them interested. I started James off at about fifteen months with some simple biscuits and then a few cakes – he is already showing a lot of interest in cooking and loves to help mother with whatever she is doing.

There are some recipes for sweet things in the preceding chapter on party food but here are some of our tried and trusty favourites that we make together in the kitchen, sometimes for desserts, some for weekends or holidays and others for when friends are visiting or we are supplying cakes for money-raising activities – which all clubs, schools and churches often have nowadays.

When your youngsters are first starting out in the kitchen I think that the nicest thing you can do is to buy them their own little apron – then it makes it a special activity when you both put on your pinnies to start cooking. You must of course teach them always to wash their hands before they start and make sure that they can safely work at the same level as yourself.

Let them start by pouring in liquids and adding items you have weighed and let them progress to being able to mix dishes and weigh items themselves. I really look forward to the day when James can make something completely by himself from start to finish – it will be a very proud moment.

Biscuits

Although I am happy for my two to have a biscuit when they are at toddlers' clubs or round at friends' houses, unless we have guests we do not resort to biscuits at home. They are both perfectly happy to be given fresh fruit as snacks and if mother is worried that they have not eaten enough at lunchtime to see them through the afternoon, then I would give them some cheese and crackers or tiny sandwiches to tide them over. In the summer months we made use of scones and little currant buns which are substantial without being too sugary.

However, biscuits and cakes are great fun to make with your toddler and they don't have to eat them all themselves – hand them out to friends, or give daddy a treat when he gets home. And above all when they have had sugary foods make sure that they brush their teeth. You can register your child with the dentist even before they have teeth (Helena started going at six months), so get your child into the routine of regular check-ups. Sugar might not be good for them, but you can minimise its effects.

Peanut crumblies
Makes 16–20 biscuits

100g (4 oz) butter, softened
100g (4 oz) smooth peanut butter
100g (4 oz) soft brown sugar
200g (8 oz) plain flour

Pre-heat the oven to 190°C/375°F/Gas 5. Cream together the butters and sugar until fluffy. Stir in the flour and mix to a dough using 1–2 teaspoons of water to help. Take small pieces of dough, roll into little balls and place these on two non-stick baking sheets. Using a dampened fork flatten each ball into a biscuit (but don't stick them to the baking sheets). Bake for about 15 minutes until brown and transfer carefully to a wire rack to cool.

Oat and cinnamon crunchies
Makes 16–20 biscuits

100g (4 oz) butter, softened
50g (2 oz) soft brown sugar
half a teaspoon (2.5ml) ground cinnamon
100g (4 oz) plain flour
100g (4 oz) porridge oats

Pre-heat the oven to 190°C/375°F/Gas 5. Cream together the butter and sugar until fluffy. Mix in the ground cinnamon, flour and oats. Use your hands to knead into a dough adding 1–2 teaspoons of cold water to help. Take little bits of the dough, roll into little balls and place these well apart on two non-stick baking sheets. Using a dampened fork, flatten each ball into a biscuit (but making sure that they don't stick to the baking sheets). Bake for 15–20 minutes until starting to colour. Transfer carefully to a wire rack to cool.

Old-fashioned biscuits
Makes about 20

A long, long time ago I learnt to make biscuits, but I have to admit that until I had children it was not something that I had done very often. Nowadays, however, it seems to be becoming a weekly event as James is very interested in how many variations we can make from our basic biscuit recipe.

> 100g (4 oz) margarine or butter
> 100g (4 oz) caster sugar
> 1 medium egg, separated
> 200g (8 oz) plain flour
> grated rind of 1 lemon
> a little caster sugar for sprinkling

Pre-heat the oven to 200°C/400°F/Gas 6. Cream together the butter and sugar until fluffy. Add the egg yolk and beat well. Sift in the flour and stir in the grated lemon rind. Knead to a dough (use a tiny amount of milk if your mixture seems too firm to handle). Place on a floured surface and roll out fairly thinly. Cut out your biscuits using any shaped cutters that you have. Place on non-stick baking sheets and bake for 10 minutes. Brush with lightly beaten egg white and sprinkle with a little caster sugar. Return to the oven for another 5–10 minutes until a pale golden brown.

Orange biscuits

Replace the lemon with the grated rind of an orange.

Vanilla biscuits

Replace the lemon with a few drops of vanilla extract.

Spiced biscuits

Replace the lemon with 1 teaspoon (5ml) mixed spice and 1 teaspoon (5ml) ground cinnamon.

Easter biscuits

Make as for the spiced biscuits but also add 2 tablespoons (30ml) currants and 1 tablespoon (15ml) chopped mixed peel.

Shrewsbury biscuits

To the old-fashioned biscuit mixture add 2 tablespoons (30ml) currants.

Muesli munchies
Makes 26–30

For a more modern, more 'health-conscious' snack (especially good for picnics or lunchboxes) try one of these.

    150g (6 oz) soft margarine
    100g (4 oz) soft brown sugar
    1 medium egg, lightly beaten
    150g (6 oz) self-raising flour
    150g (6 oz) no-added-sugar muesli

Pre-heat the oven to 180°C/350°F/Gas 4. Cream the margarine and sugar together until fluffy. Beat in the egg and then stir in the flour and muesli. Mix well and place in little mounds on lightly greased baking sheets – leave room for the munchies to expand. Bake in the pre-heated oven for 10–15 minutes until golden brown. Transfer carefully to a wire rack to cool.

Small cakes

Young children always seem to particularly enjoy making these sorts of cakes – I know I can still remember helping to lay out the paper cases when I was a child. I have used the basic recipe for fairy cakes, or cupcakes as we used to call them, from the chapter on party food – but here is a special recipe for chocolate fairy or 'butterfly' cakes which is absolutely delicious and very popular with my son James and his friends.

Chocolate fairy cakes
Makes 16

> 100g (4 oz) soft margarine
> 100g (4 oz) caster sugar
> 2 medium eggs, lightly beaten
> 75g (3 oz) self-raising flour
> 25g (1 oz) cocoa powder
> 1 teaspoon (5ml) baking powder
>
> *Chocolate buttercream*
> 3 tablespoons (45ml) hot water
> 2 tablespoons (30ml) cocoa powder
> 150g (6 oz) butter, softened
> 300g (12 oz) icing sugar, sifted

Pre-heat the oven to 200°C/400°F/Gas 6. Cream together the soft margarine and the sugar until fluffy, beat in the eggs, self-raising flour, the cocoa and the baking powder. Divide 16 paper cases between 2 baking sheets and divide the mixture between these. Bake in the pre-heated oven for 15–20 minutes until well risen. Cool on a wire rack. To make the chocolate buttercream, mix together the hot water and cocoa powder to a thick cream and leave to cool slightly. Then beat together with the softened butter and sifted icing sugar. (It is important to sift the icing sugar or you will have lumps in the buttercream.) Cut a small slice from the top of each cake and cut this circle in half. Put some buttercream on the top of each cake and then arrange the two circle halves as 'wings' on top.

Apart from all the different types of fairy cakes that we make the other small cakes that we like to make are scones, rock cakes, madeleines, muffins and a number of very tasty traybakes.

Scones

Fruit scones
Makes 12

>   200g (8 oz) self-raising flour
>   2 teaspoons (10ml) baking powder
>   50g (2 oz) butter or margarine
>   50g (2 oz) currants
>   25g (1 oz) caster sugar
>   125ml (5 fl oz) milk
>   extra milk for glazing

Pre-heat the oven to 220°C/425°F/Gas 7. Put the flour, baking powder and butter or margarine into a bowl and using your fingertips rub the mixture together until it resembles breadcrumbs. Stir in the currants and caster sugar. Add enough of the milk to give a firm dough. On a floured surface roll out the dough to about 3cm (1 inch) thick and cut out little rounds with a scone cutter. Place on a lightly greased baking sheet and brush with milk. Bake in the pre-heated oven for 10–12 minutes or until risen and brown. Cool on a wire rack.

Cheese scones
Makes 12

200g (8 oz) self-raising flour
2 teaspoons (10ml) baking powder
pinch of salt
50g (2 oz) butter or margarine
75g (3 oz) grated cheddar cheese
pinch of dry English mustard
1 egg, beaten and made up to 125ml (5 fl oz) with
   milk
extra milk for glazing

Pre-heat the oven to 220°C/425°F/Gas 7. Place the flour, baking powder, salt and butter or margarine in a bowl and using your fingertips rub the ingredients together until you have a breadcrumb-like mixture. Stir in the cheddar cheese and the dry mustard and then use enough of the milk and egg mixture to get a firm dough. Roll out on a floured surface to about 3cm (1 inch) thick and using a scone cutter cut out your scones. Place on a lightly greased baking sheet, glaze with milk and bake in the pre-heated oven for 10–12 minutes until risen and brown. Cool on a wire rack.

Rock cakes
Makes 8–12

I have used white self-raising flour in this recipe but you can make it just as well with the same amount of wholemeal self-raising flour or a mixture of half and half. Also you can vary the sugar that you use – try caster sugar, soft dark brown sugar or light muscovado sugar. For the mixed dried fruit try using a luxury mix or make your own mix from the many types of ready-to-eat dried fruits that are now available. Both sultana and apricot and sultana and pineapple have proved to be very popular in our household.

200g (8 oz) self-raising flour
2 teaspoons (10ml) baking powder
1 teaspoon (5ml) mixed spice
100g (4 oz) margarine
grated rind of half a lemon (optional)
100g (4 oz) demerara sugar
100g (4 oz) mixed dried fruit
1 egg, lightly beaten
1–2 tablespoons (15–30ml) milk
extra demerara

Pre-heat the oven to 200°C/400°F/Gas 6. Rub together the flour, baking powder, mixed spice and margarine to a crumb-like mixture. Stir in the other ingredients, using enough milk to give you a stiff mixture. Place the mixture in small dollops on lightly greased baking trays. Sprinkle with extra demerara sugar. Bake for 15–20 minutes until golden then transfer to a wire rack to cool.

Madeleines
Makes 8–10

These are a great favourite with the children. They aren't bothered about eating them, but they do love making them – even Helena can help to decorate them.

100g (4 oz) butter
100g (4 oz) caster sugar
2 eggs, lightly beaten
100g (4 oz) self raising flour

to decorate
glace cherries, halved
raspberry or strawberry jam
desiccated coconut

Pre-heat the oven to 180°C/350°F/Gas 4. Cream together the butter and sugar, and then beat in the eggs and fold in the flour. Half fill lightly greased dariole moulds with the mixture and place on a baking tray. Bake in the pre-heated oven for about 20 minutes until well risen and golden brown. Cool in the moulds for 5 minutes and then turn out onto a wire rack to cool completely. Then comes the fun part. Melt the jam (the children enjoy sieving the seeds out – but make sure that the jam is cool enough for them), brush the jam over the madeleines and then roll in the coconut (this is messy when the children do it!). Top each madeleine with half a cherry.

PS If you don't have dariole moulds, put the mixture into paper cases and when cooked, decorate the tops with jam, coconut and halved cherries.

Coconut Pyramids
Makes approx. 18

To make these you need a little pyramid-shaped object that has a plunger that extricates the mixture as a little pyramid. You could just make little heaps of the mixture, but using this strange object is half the fun. You can obtain them from Lakeland Plastics.

200g (8 oz) desiccated coconut
100g (4 oz) caster sugar
2 egg whites, beaten

Pre-heat the oven to 180°C/350°F/Gas 4. Cover two baking trays with baking parchment. Mix together the coconut and sugar and use enough of the beaten egg white to bind stiffly together. Pack mixture into pyramid maker and release onto baking parchment (or just put in little heaps on the paper). Continue until mixture is all used. Bake for 15–20 minutes until a pale golden brown. Cool on a wire rack.

Muffins

These have only really become popular in this country in the last decade, and as I had not come across them in my cookery classes at school, it was a while before I started to experiment with them – and I'm still learning as I go. Although similar to our fairy cakes, the principles in cooking them are quite different, the main problem being that if overmixed they become very rubbery. However, once you have got the knack of really just 'throwing' them together then they really are very easy to make – and I suspect that muffins are very easy for those who are new to baking as they don't make the mistake of trying to get a perfect mixture. Muffin tins and papers are widely available in large and small sizes. Although the small ones are perfect for small children I have found the larger ones just as popular as, although too big for many children to eat a whole one, most just like the feel of them in their hands and like taking little bites out of them. Muffins make a great breakfast treat.

Although muffins do not keep very well – they are really best eaten on the day they are made, and I would never keep them for more than a day or two – they do freeze well. Make sure that you wrap them well, then when you want to use them either defrost a couple of hours beforehand or overnight, then a quick burst in the

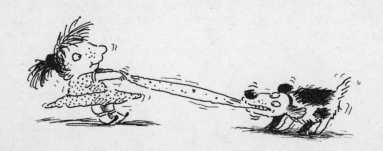

oven or microwave will heat them through perfectly.

The amount of batter to make six large muffins should make about eighteen small muffins but the smaller ones will cook in about fifteen to twenty minutes.

Blueberry muffins
Makes 12 large muffins

> 250g (10 oz) plain flour
> 4 teaspoons (20ml) baking powder
> pinch of ground cinnamon
> grated rind of 1 lemon
> 75g (3 oz) caster sugar
> 2 medium eggs, beaten
> 50g (2 oz) butter, melted
> 200ml (8 fl oz) milk
> 225g (9 oz) fresh blueberries
> little extra flour
> 1 tablespoon (15ml) demerara sugar

Pre-heat the oven to 200°C/400°F/Gas 6. Place 12 large muffin cases in muffin tins. In a large bowl mix together the plain flour, baking powder, cinnamon, grated lemon rind and the sugar. In a separate bowl, mix together the eggs, melted butter (but this should not be hot) and the milk. Quickly mix into the dry ingredients. Do not overmix – the mixture should be lumpy. Sprinkle the blueberries with about a tablespoon (15ml) of flour and mix well (this makes sure that they don't just sink to the bottom of the batter) and then quickly fold into the batter. Divide the batter between the muffin cases and sprinkle with the demerara sugar. Bake for 20–25 minutes until well risen and firm to the touch. Cool a little on a wire rack. Serve warm.

Other great flavour combinations we have made using this recipe include banana, substituting chopped banana for the blueberries; apple, replacing the fruit with two grated apples; and apricot, substituting ready-to-eat dried chopped apricots.

Double choc chip muffins
Makes 6 large muffins

100g (4 oz) plain flour
25g (1 oz) cocoa powder
1 dessertspoon (10ml) baking powder
40g (1½ oz) caster sugar
1 medium egg, beaten
half a teaspoon (2.5ml) vanilla extract
25g (1 oz) butter, melted (but not hot)
100ml (4 fl oz) milk
100g (4 oz) plain chocolate chips

Pre-heat the oven to 200°C/400°F/Gas 6. Place 6 large muffin cases in a muffin tin. In a large bowl mix together the plain flour, cocoa powder, baking powder and the sugar. In a separate bowl mix together the beaten egg, vanilla extract, melted butter and the milk. Now quickly mix the dry and wet ingredients together. Do not overmix, the batter should be lumpy. Fold in the chocolate chips and divide the batter between the cases. Cook in the pre-heated oven for 20–25 minutes until well risen and firm to the touch. Transfer to a wire rack to cool slightly. Serve just warm.

Maple and raisin muffins
Makes 6 large muffins

125g (5 oz) plain flour
1 tablespoon (15ml) baking powder
2 tablespoons (30ml) maple syrup
1 medium egg, lightly beaten
25g (1 oz) butter, melted (but not hot)
100ml (4 fl oz) milk
100g (4 oz) raisins
1 tablespoon (15ml) demerara sugar

Pre-heat the oven to 200°C/400°F/Gas 6. Put 6 muffin papers in a 6-hole muffin tin. Mix together the plain flour and baking powder in a large bowl. In a separate bowl mix together the maple syrup, beaten egg, melted butter and milk. Quickly mix in with the dry ingredients – do not overmix, you should have a lumpy consistency. Fold the raisins into the batter. Divide the batter between the muffin cases and sprinkle with the demerara sugar. Bake in the pre-heated oven for 20–25 minutes until well risen and brown. Serve warm.

Traybakes

These are easy to mix and bake and are very useful for picnics and for producing for sales, etc. Divide into suitable portions for your purpose – usually around twelve.

Flapjacks

These are probably the cakes that I have made most often – now that we have children I am making them just a touch softer. Now I sometimes make them with raisins or chocolate chips as well (I add about 100g (4 oz) of these when using). If adding chocolate chips to the flapjack mixture, let the mixture cool before stirring them in or they will just melt. With flapjacks it is important not to overbake them, or they will turn out hard.

    150g (6 oz) butter or margarine
    150g (6 oz) soft dark brown sugar
    1 tablespoon (15ml) golden syrup
    225g (9 oz) porridge oats

Pre-heat the oven to 170°C/325°F/Gas 3. Put the butter or margarine, the sugar and golden syrup in a saucepan and heat gently until the mixture melts. Remove from the heat and stir in the oats. Mix well and then press into a lightly greased 18 × 28cm (7 × 11 inch) baking tin. Bake in the pre-heated oven for 20 minutes until pale golden brown. Leave to cool for a few minutes, then mark into portions. Leave to cool completely in the tin.

Iced lemon cake

200g (8 oz) self-raising flour
150g (6 oz) soft margarine
150g (6 oz) caster sugar
2 teaspoons (10ml) baking powder
grated rind of 1 lemon
3 eggs
3 tablespoons (45ml) milk

Lemon glacé icing
150g (6oz) icing sugar, sifted
2–3 tablespoons (30–45ml) juice from the lemon

Pre-heat the oven to 180°C/350°F/Gas 4. Grease and line an 18 × 28cm (7 × 11 inch) baking tin. Put all the ingredients for the cake in a large bowl and beat well. Turn into the baking tin and level the top. Bake in the pre-heated oven for 30–35 minutes until it is golden brown, 'springy' to the touch and has shrunk slightly from the sides of the tin. Leave to cool completely in the tin. Mix the icing sugar with enough lemon juice to get a thick but runny consistency and spread over the top of the cake. Leave to set. Cut into portions to serve.

Coffee and pecan bake

Don't make the mistake of thinking that you must always add a topping to bakes – although I have given a recipe for coffee icing to top this one, we often omit it as James loves this cake so much he starts picking at it before we get a chance to ice it!

200g (8 oz) self-raising flour
150g (6 oz) light muscovado sugar
150g (6 oz) soft margarine
2 teaspoons (10ml) baking powder
3 eggs
2 tablespoons (30ml) milk
1 tablespoon (15ml) coffee essence
50g (2 oz) pecans, ground (or very finely chopped)

Coffee icing
150g (6 oz) icing sugar, sifted
50g (2 oz) butter
2 teaspoons (10ml) milk
1 teaspoon (5ml) coffee essence

Pre-heat the oven to 180°C/350°F/Gas 4. Grease and line an 18 × 28cm (7 × 11 inch) baking tin. Place all the cake ingredients in a large bowl and beat well. Turn into the prepared tin and level the top. Bake in the pre-heated oven for 30–35 minutes or until the bake is golden brown, 'springy' to the touch and shrinks slightly from the sides of the tin. Cool in the tin. To make the coffee icing, beat together the sifted icing sugar, butter, milk and coffee essence. Spread roughly over the bake and leave to set. Divide into portions before serving.

Sultana and apricot bake

150g (6 oz) self-raising flour
150g (6 oz) caster sugar
150g (6 oz) soft margarine
50g (2 oz) ground almonds
2 teaspoons (10ml) baking powder
3 eggs
3 tablespoons (45ml) milk
75g (3 oz) sultanas
75g (3 oz) ready-to-eat dried apricots, chopped
demerara sugar to decorate

Pre-heat the oven to 180°C/350°F/Gas 4. Grease and line an 18 × 28cm (7 × 11 inch) baking tray. Place all the cake ingredients in a large bowl and beat well. Turn into the prepared tin and bake in the pre-heated oven for 20 minutes. Sprinkle with demerara sugar and then bake for a further 10 minutes or until the cake is 'springy' and has shrunk a little from the sides of the tin. Cool in the tin. Divide into portions before serving.

Fruitcake bake

200g (8 oz) self-raising wholemeal flour
150g (6 oz) muscovado sugar
150g (6 oz) soft margarine
2 teaspoons (10ml) baking powder
1 teaspoon (5ml) ground cinnamon
3 eggs
3 tablespoons (45ml) milk
250g (10 oz) luxury fruit mix
100g (4 oz) glacé cherries, chopped
demerara sugar

Pre-heat the oven to 170°C/325°F/Gas 3. Grease and line an 18 × 28cm (7 × 11 inch) baking tin. In a large bowl beat together the flour, sugar, margarine, baking powder, cinnamon, eggs and milk. Stir in the fruit mix and chopped cherries. Turn into the prepared baking tin and cook for 30 minutes. Sprinkle with the demerara sugar and cook for a further 20–25 minutes until firm to the touch and the cake has shrunk away slightly from the sides of the tin. Leave to cool in the tin. Divide into portions to serve.

Desserts

Although in our household (and in most households with small children) dessert is usually some fruit or a yoghurt, we do occasionally indulge in a sweet dessert. This tends to be for a weekend lunch or a holiday treat. Nine times out of ten these desserts will be fruit based – we do like fruit in our house!

In the summer we tend to go for freshly picked fruit served with cream, custard or home-made ice-cream. In the autumn and winter months it will often be turned into a fruit crumble. Our other firm family favourites are trifles and fools. Asking around other families I found that trifle was a big hit with other youngsters as well – just be careful not to make it with as much alcohol as you would normally!

Family trifle
Makes 6–8 adult portions

This is a very simple recipe for trifle, which is just how our two like it. You can of course add some chopped jelly at the same time as adding the fruit or split the trifle sponges and sandwich together with some jam – the recipe is very elastic.

    6–8 trifle sponges
    125ml (5 fl oz) orange juice, medium sherry or a
      mixture of both
    300–400g (12–16 oz) fresh or canned fruit
    500ml (1 pint) custard
    250ml (10 fl oz) whipping cream, lightly whipped
    fresh fruit to decorate

Put enough trifle sponges in your trifle bowl to completely cover the bottom of the bowl. Soak with the orange juice or sherry. Cover with your chosen fruit. Now spoon the custard over the fruit and leave to set. Cover the custard with the whipping cream and decorate with slices of fruit.

Fruit crumble
Makes 4–6 adult portions

If you are using fresh berry fruit you will have little preparation. However, if you are using apples I prefer to cook them quickly in a tablespoon of soft margarine or butter for just a few minutes before mixing them with the sugar and putting in the pie dish. Rhubarb needs no pre-cooking, just cutting into suitable lengths. For a very tart fruit such as gooseberries I would add a little more sugar. I sometimes add a little juice to some fruits, for example a little orange juice to rhubarb, or a little elderflower cordial to gooseberries. I have just discovered that both James and Helena are particularly fond of apple and elderflower. So do ring the changes – I'm sure that if you had a crumble every weekend throughout the year you would not have to repeat the same recipe twice. You can also play around with the crumble topping, adding oats or cereals. I have also found that polenta and semolina make good additions.

1kg (2 lb) prepared fruit
2 tablespoons (30ml) caster sugar

Crumble topping
100g (4 oz) self-raising flour
100g (4 oz) caster sugar
100g (4 oz) butter, chopped

Pre-heat the oven to 200°C/400°F/Gas 6. Mix the prepared fruit with the 2 tablespoons of caster sugar and put into a pie dish. Using the tips of your fingers, rub together the flour, sugar and butter until you have a crumb-like topping. Completely cover the fruit with the crumble topping. Bake in the pre-heated oven for 30 minutes until brown.

Fruit fools

Basically these are stewed or puréed fruits mixed with yoghurt or custard and cream. As a rough quantity guide, allow about 50–100g (2–4 oz) of fruit for children and double this amount for adults. For fruits such as rhubarb and gooseberries, add 1 tablespoon of caster sugar per 500g (1lb) of fruit and stew very gently for about 15 minutes. For fruit with stones you will also have to add 1–2 tablespoons (15–30ml) of water per 500g (1lb) of fruit. (Remove the stones after stewing.) Purée the fruit and measure how much you have. You will want an equal amount of yoghurt or custard and cream. I usually make my fools with half as much cream as the amount of yoghurt I am using, so the resulting fool is three parts fruit purée, two parts yoghurt or custard and one part cream. To make the fool mix your fruit purée with yoghurt (Greek style is lovely) or custard to make a creamy mixture. Add a touch of honey if it seems a little sharp. Then lightly whip some whipping cream and fold it into the fruit mixture. Chill well before serving and serve with some little sweet biscuits for dipping.

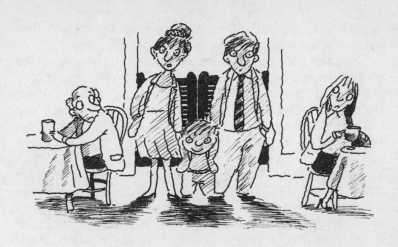

10. Eating out

When you first embark on parenthood it can often seem like your social life has come to an end, that those days of casually deciding to go out for a meal or a trip to the pub have come abruptly to a halt. You may even decide that with all the new expenses you are incurring you will never be able to afford a social life again. However, you quickly realise that in order to save your sanity you really must get out of the house. And whatever the effort involved in doing so and even if the trip didn't last very long, the important factor is that you did it – you managed to achieve what only a little while ago seemed like an impossible task. The first outing we had with James was a very quick foray to our local pub. All we wanted was one drink in civilised surroundings – luckily we're fast drinkers, because it wasn't long before we were forced home by a screaming baby. But how good it felt just to sit in the sun, in what seemed like another world, sipping our drinks – it was as if screaming babies didn't exist. So although it was only a brief experience, we had done it and we had glimpsed that maybe there was going to be life after children.

Over the past three years we have had the chance to try out many eating places with either James, Helena or the two of them. Certainly as they get older it does become a little easier. There are certain ages that are easier to cope with. For instance, newborns may be very difficult to accommodate but once they have got into the swing of sleeping and eating at certain times you may well be able to arrange trips out with very little trouble (especially if mother is breastfeeding, so there is no need to worry about heating bottles). However, when you start to wean your baby, you may begin to hit a few problems – unless you take your own baby food with you – as many places will not cater for young babies. Then again when baby is on the move, this provides plenty of scope for problems for parents. If you want to have any chance of enjoying your meal then you must have somewhere to 'tether' your baby. Once your child is eating the same meals as the rest of the family, going out to eat does become so much easier. The main problems are now keeping them amused – quick service is a definite plus at this point. Long leisurely meals are out.

So once your children are able to eat a wide variety of food, can go to the toilet and can be trusted to sit quietly for a reasonable length of time or amuse themselves without disturbing you or your fellow diners, you will be able to return to a civilised way of life. At the moment this is still some way in the future for us – we are just happy to get out sometimes. It may not exactly be restful but it does make for a break from routine and the children enjoy it greatly.

I have compiled a list of places that we have taken our children to and said how successful these trips have been. It is in no way a comprehensive list, it reflects where we live (in the south east of England) and have travelled with the children (up to Scotland, through parts of Yorkshire, the Lake District, down to Land's End in Cornwall, and Paris). I cannot comment on places we have not been to, but hope that this list may give you some ideas of places to visit and have a fairly pleasurable meal with your children.

We consider that the basic minimum requirement that must be met when out with a baby is that the venue can either heat a baby's bottle or heat up baby food or provide you with hot water. For very young children quick service is important or you are going to have trouble on your hands. Service can vary greatly and when you visit may be a big factor in this respect, so choose your time wisely.

If you visit somewhere with only the basic minimum of facilities for children then you will often find that what makes or mars your trip will be the attitude of the staff – this can make up for the lack of many facilities.

Many places nowadays have started to cater for young children, providing highchairs, changing facilities, baby food, and making efforts to amuse the children – some provide crayons and a colouring sheet, and some even provide play areas. Again the attitude of the staff can make such a big difference. So in my list, as well as saying what is generally provided, I have indicated how successful the trip was with a smiling face – one indicates a bare minimum was achieved to three to indicate that all the stops were pulled out. Two faces plus (+) is not quite as good as three.

Ideas for eating out with your children

Granny's ☺ ☺ ☺

This must depend on your particular parents – but for most people is hard to beat. You may have to provide some of the facilities yourself or some guidance on what food to provide, but whatever facilities may be lacking, grandparents can make up for in keeping the children amused. Highly recommended for long weekends or when husbands are away on business trips.

Meals at friends' houses ☺ ☺ ☺

A very popular option especially if they have children of their own, as the children will hopefully amuse each other. There are different toys to play with and like-minded adults to talk to. If your friends don't have children one drawback may be that the house is not child proof and you will spend a lot of time preventing your children from demolishing the house. The plus point is that your friends must love you a lot to invite you and your brood into their nice clean child-free zone!

TGI Fridays ☺ ☺ ☺

Very, very good – if they only provided small play areas they would be absolutely unbeatable. They provided a highchair, good changing facilities, free baby food, pre-wrapped feeding spoon, crackers for baby to chew on, they can heat bottles, the service was impeccable, and they will do juggling or other tricks to amuse the children. Balloons, crayons and colouring sheets provided for everyone, soft drinks are refilled free (this is something that is commonplace in the United States and really should catch on here) and the choice of food was good. These people are trying to please – let's hope that one day there will be a lot more like them.

Chef and Brewer's Wacky Warehouses ☺ ☺ +

Although not all Chef and Brewers have these Wacky Warehouses, the ones that do are very good. They will provide you with hot water with which to heat up bottles and baby food, we have found the staff to be very helpful and the children have indoor and outdoor playing areas (although the indoor ones are geared towards payment – but the money goes to children's charities). Plenty of highchairs and the service is generally good. (You order at counters and the food is brought to you.) The choice of food is very good, the specials of the day often include fresh seasonal produce made in a home-cooked style – we've had some very good meals there. How good they are may depend on individual chefs. Get there early as this chain is very popular.

Happy Eaters ☺ ☺ +

When travelling, unless picnicking, we always aim to stop off for meal breaks here. Bottles can be heated, baby food provided, there are high chairs and crayons and colouring sheets. The service is generally quick and best of all there are often indoor and outdoor playing areas. There is a reasonable choice of food which has improved over the last year or so. Some are definitely excellent – a lot can depend on individual staff and how busy they are. We've sometimes had problems getting James to leave!

Supermarkets ☺ ☺ +

The big supermarkets with coffee shops attached are very good. They have good changing facilities, provide highchairs, bottles can be warmed and at most baby food can be purchased or is provided free. The service is quick and a reasonable choice of food is offered. We have been to two Safeway stores which also have play areas for children, a trend which I hope catches on as more superstores are built.

Airports ☺ ☺

We live close to Heathrow and Gatwick and on a rainy day I have entertained the children by visiting Gatwick Airport. There is a small train that they love, many shops and a tiny play area. The cafés have the same facilities as the average café but the airport itself has better facilities. When actually travelling by air, we are spoilt as, because of the amount of travelling involved in Andy's job, he (and us when travelling with him) can use the executive lounges. This makes life a lot easier as the facilities are less crowded (we were lucky as when we were travelling with friends, we had a small room with a video and a train set which was just being used by our children) and checking in is easier. Travelling by air with small children is not really my idea of fun. The airlines do try but although slightly older children should enjoy it, very little children are soon bored. However, if you are travelling by air, they will be able to heat the baby's milk, and should supply small children with crayons, etc. The cabin staff will try to be helpful, but they are generally very busy.

Burger chains ☺ ☺

The good points about these are that service is very quick, that highchairs are provided and that they can heat babies' bottles. They just creep out of the basic category because they also sometimes provide colouring sheets or balloons and they appear on most high streets. However, the choice of food provided leaves a lot to be desired!

Children's farms ☺ ☺

These are increasingly popular and we are lucky to have a couple of really good ones near us. You will find a lot of difference in the facilities, but all should be able to warm a baby's bottle. At some you can buy baby food, at others the food on offer is very limited (just cakes, etc.). Some will have highchairs. At most the staff are extremely friendly. The best have good play areas (both in and out) and the children love the animals.

Department stores, high street shops with restaurants ☺ ☺

Many big high street stores have a little restaurant in them – BHS, Boots, Littlewoods, etc. These will have highchairs and should heat up baby food and bottles for you. Changing facilities are generally good and the range of food offered should be good. Helpful staff are what really make the difference here and I must praise our Debenhams store as the service here is always first class.

Harvester ☺ ☺

Again when travelling or going out for a Sunday lunch this is a popular choice with us. They have highchairs and will heat baby food and bottles for you. We love the salad bar and picking at this keeps Helena amused for ages. We have generally found the service to be good and the staff to be really helpful (many are mums themselves) so this is a good choice.

Motorway services ☺ ☺

Again they vary enormously but you should have no problems in getting bottles or baby food heated. Some do have baby food for sale, but don't rely on it. Highchairs and changing facilities should be good. Some have play areas. We have found some food to be really good, others quite poor. The choice is slowly but surely improving.

Picnics in parks, etc. ☺ ☺

The success of these outings will depend on your forethought and the weather! We've had some really lovely picnics with our two, and all through winter James has been talking about the summer and it being picnic time again. The two main drawbacks are that parents with young children will probably not get much rest as once out of the pushchair the baby is off, and has to be retrieved again and again! The other drawback can be toilet facilities for newly toilet-trained youngsters. This option has a lot of pros, however, on the cost side.

Swimming pools, leisure facilities ☺ ☺

Again a wide variance but generally the more modern the facility the better equipped for children it will be. The good eating areas will usually be poolside with highchairs and a reasonable choice of food. Service should be quick and they will be able to heat babies' bottles for you. The attitude of the staff is generally friendly. Again we are very lucky as we have two very good pools within twenty minutes of us. We also found an excellent one on holiday in Scotland which the children greatly enjoyed and which gave us something to do on a rainy day (in Scotland – never!).

Theme parks, zoos, etc. ☺ ☺

Very hard to generalise but the facilities are generally good as, although often aimed at older children, some thought has gone into facilities for younger children too. Most have a wide range of food outlets so you should have a reasonable choice. Highchairs are commonplace and many have good changing facilities and often play areas. Not all will provide baby food, but you should be able to heat babies' bottles or baby food. Some will be excellent but all should have reasonable facilities. Larger theme parks on the whole will have better or more refined facilities.

We've particularly enjoyed Legoland, Monkeyworld, Crinkly Bottom, Paultons and Marwell Zoo. Legoland was wonderful; we spent six hours there and we've never spent that long anywhere with our two children. Monkeyworld, although being small and having few facilities, had a fantastic range of healthy sandwiches (in an area which seems to thrive on fried foods) and the monkey nursery has a glass wall dividing the big soft area where your children can play from the baby monkeys, all this where parents can sit relaxing with their meals – wonderful.

Warehouse stores with restaurant facilities – IKEA, etc. ☺ ☺

These will vary but many are quite well thought out – some do provide play areas, for example. We liked our local IKEA. Highchairs were provided, the changing facilities were good and there were microwave ovens which could be used to heat baby food, etc. Also there was a small playing area in the restaurant. There is a reasonable choice of food. (Helena had her very first chip here, which she stole from her brother's plate before we realised she could reach it.)

Cafés and coffee shops ☺ +

A huge variance, but you should be able to get bottles heated up for your baby. Many have highchairs, but certainly not all. The attitude of the staff and how busy they are will certainly play a big part in your visit. Many staff in small coffee shops will be enormously friendly and helpful (again they're often mums themselves).

Pizza places ☺

These do vary quite a lot and some are more geared up towards children than others. On the whole though all you will get here is the baby's bottle warmed up and a highchair. More popular with older children.

Pubs ☺

Perhaps I am being a little unfair here but certainly the average pub does not cater for children and certainly its biggest drawback is changing/toilet facilities for young children. We have been to ordinary pubs that provide highchairs for children (generally when in a tourist area) but these are few and far between. In some pubs the choice of food can be very good; in others it is atrocious. Service again can vary enormously. This is one instance where the attitude of the staff will make or mar your visit. We've had some great meals at pubs, even where there were no facilities but where the staff were so helpful that it didn't matter. You will have more luck if you visit on a sunny day and can sit in the garden or if the pub has a family room.

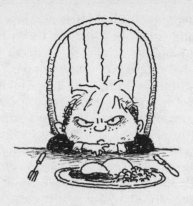

11. Mother's worst fear – the difficult eater!

What do you do when your darling child refuses to eat your humble offerings? The answer is that in reality there really is very little you can do. I know that some people say you should arrange the food on the plate in a child-friendly manner, dressing it up as a clown's face, etc. But in my experience this doesn't work. If a child wants to eat something then he will, if he doesn't want to eat it then he won't. The sooner that parents accept this the easier life will be. The exceptions to this are when a child is refusing food because he is really tired, is feeling unwell, or is not really hungry when the food is offered to him. Then if you can remedy the situation you will often find that the food that was being refused will be eaten.

The absolute worst scenario is a child that constantly refuses to try any new foods. There really are many children like this and most go through a stage of behaving in this way – so don't worry, your child is completely normal and you are doing nothing wrong.

It is heartbreaking to spend time and money on meals for your children and then to see them being wasted, but at the end of the day if they don't want it, they won't eat it. Although you may be worried that your child is not eating enough or not having a healthy balanced diet, it is amazing how little food children can actually exist on, and you can always supplement their diet with vitamin drops if you really are worried. If you become concerned that your child really seems to be eating nothing at all over a period of weeks, then contact your health visitor for reassurance. Maybe there is a medical reason and your child should be checked over – however, this is unlikely if the child appears well and is active and happy in himself. James has in the past gone for a period of six weeks hardly eating anything, but then suddenly reverted back to his normal eating pattern.

If you are concerned that your child is really putting on too much weight, check this out with your health visitor before trying to do anything about it. Again there could be a medical reason behind this or your child may naturally have a bigger build than other children you are comparing him to. However, if it is just that your child is consuming too many calories then you can easily switch his diet to accommodate this. Cutting down on fatty and sugary foods and increasing the fruit and vegetables in his diet should be all you need to do.

What is important when you have a child who is a very finicky eater is to continue to offer the foods that you want him to eat – if you never offer them the child can never accept them. You can also try disguising certain foods by putting them in soups, sauces, etc. – this does sometimes work. But I would never force food on any child. Don't offer a type of food that has been rejected too often, just occasionally to see if they have changed their mind, and offer it in different forms. My two will not eat eggs, whether boiled, scrambled, fried or as omelettes, but they do consume cakes and custard made with eggs. They obviously really dislike the taste of 'egg'. Sometimes it is the texture of a dish that your child dislikes.

Do make sure that you keep portion sizes small initially; nothing puts most children off faster than a plate piled with food. So keep portions small and only increase them when your child is clearing his plate. If your child shows a preference for certain vegetables, give him a little more next time and less of ones that he leaves. Don't be surprised when he suddenly goes off food that he normally loves, or when he constantly asks for a certain food, but when you serve it barely touches it. This is perfectly normal behaviour in small children.

The one thing that you should not do is to make a scene when food is refused. And this is so difficult to do in practice! Just try, try and try to keep calm, because anger will only provoke your child into a battle of wills.

If your child is constantly refusing foods, it is doubly important not to spend too much time and energy on a pointless exercise – you will gradually just make yourself feel worse and worse and will achieve nothing. Simplify your meals as much as possible. Base them on foods that your child will eat and are easy to prepare, then gradually add other foods, but don't insist that they are eaten. Do not let your child fill up on snacks that have no nutritional value, and make sure that they are not filling themselves up with liquids. Ensure that all the drinks they do have are nutritional in themselves – milk, milkshakes made with real fruit and unsweetened fruit juices all have considerable nutritional benefits.

It is extremely worrying when your child is not eating as you would wish him to, but you will be better off if you can hide your worry. It is so difficult to do, but if you can, both you and your child will be all the happier. Good luck!

Index

mince 132
sausage casserole 144
see also game
Vicarage roast 105

weaning 20, **31–50**

yoghurt 20–21, 57–8
see also menus

GRUB ON A GRANT

Cas Clarke

Cheap and Foolproof Recipes for All Students

' . . . a useful little book for an absolute beginner. My children simply loved her Varsity Pie.'
Prue Leith, *Guardian*

' . . . written by a student who experienced the problems of cooking for herself for the first time while at the University of Sussex; she reckons her recipes are foolproof, and so they are.' *Daily Telegraph*

' . . . full of extremely practical and sensible advice and some hilarious cartoons, giving an exciting repertoire of meals whatever the culinary abilities.'
Jill Probert, *Liverpool Daily Post*

Grub on a Grant found an unexpectedly large and eager market when it was first published in autumn 1985. Perhaps it struck a special chord with young people because it recognized that they are short not only of money but of time and culinary gadgetry as well – but they do like to eat well, and they especially love food with clearly identifiable flavours. For this revised and updated edition of her book Cas Clarke has greatly expanded the vegetarian section. There are also some exciting dinner party recipes and a chapter on slow cooking.

Whether you are on a student grant, unemployed or just generally impoverished, you'll find this new edition of *Grub on a Grant* a very sound investment.

NON-FICTION / COOKERY 0 7472 3560 0

More Non-Fiction from Headline

PECKISH BUT POOR

Cas Clarke

Delicious Budget Recipes by the Author of *Grub on a Grant*

Cas Clarke's *Grub on a Grant* was hugely popular with students struggling with a single saucepan and a grant. *Peckish but Poor* is for would-be cooks who are ready to move on to more adventurous cookery and want to produce tasty meals on a still restricted budget.

The emphasis here is on easy-to-follow recipes using fresh produce with chapters giving recipes for spring, summer, autumn and winter showing how simple it is to make cheap and delicious dishes by keeping to food that is in season.

If you're short of time, money or experience, you'll find the uncomplicated, no-nonsense recipes in *Peckish but Poor* a brilliant way to build your confidence in the kitchen.

GRUB ON A GRANT

' . . . a useful little book for the absolute beginner.' Prue Leith, *Guardian*

' . . . she reckons her recipes are foolproof, and so they are.' *Daily Telegraph*

NON-FICTION / COOKERY 0 7472 3937 1

Beating the Biological Clock
THE JOYS AND CHALLENGES OF LATE MOTHERHOOD

Pamela Armstrong

Babies change your life. They're hard work. They disrupt your sleep and devastate the body beautiful. So why are women leaving it later and later to have their children, when the natural difficulties of having a baby are compounded by advancing years?

There are a growing band of women in their thirties and forties who buck the trend. At the very time that most women are waving their offspring goodbye and facing an empty nest, these mature mums are putting their careers on hold and having babies.

Television presenter Pamela Armstrong, who had her first baby at forty-two, has spoken to many older mothers about the myriad trials, challenges and joys of later motherhood, and her book is packed with information and anecdotes drawn directly from the experiences of women themselves. Older mothers, with more to lose, often approach pregnancy with great zeal and commitment. They want to know everything; they want the truth and the very best for their unborn child.

The book covers everything from pre-conceptual care to the increasingly divisive issue of pre-natal diagnostic testing, and the statistical reality of handicap in later births. It reassures the older mother-to-be so that she can carry, bear and nurture her new born confident that she has made all the right choices.

NON-FICTION / SELF HELP 0 7472 5077 4

MEAN BEANS

Cheap and Easy Vegetarian Cooking by the Author of GRUB ON A GRANT

Cas Clarke

Vegetarians rejoice. *Mean Beans* from Cas Clarke, author of bestselling *Grub on a Grant*, is bursting with enterprising, appetising recipes that won't wreck your budget. If you like the idea of 'going vegetarian' but are put off by nut-cutlets, these tasty, nutritious meals show you how to eat well using fresh seasonal ingredients or raiding the store cupboard when funds run low.

Practical, straightforward and user-friendly, *Mean Beans* makes vegetarian cooking economical and easy.

'She reckons her recipes are foolproof, and so they are' *Daily Telegraph*

NON-FICTION / COOKERY 0 7472 4233 X

Vegetarian Grub on a Grant

CAS CLARKE

Since the publication, ten years ago, of Cas Clarke's hugely successful *Grub on a Grant* there has been a revolution in eating habits: lots of meat is out; vegetarian food is in. Many students recognise that a vegetarian diet is both nourishing and cheap but they need help in producing appetising meals on limited means.

Vegetarian Grub on a Grant is for everyone who is struggling with a single saucepan and a grant. Appreciating the constraints under which students cook, Cas Clarke gives masses of straightforward recipes, many of which can be prepared in a single pan. There are meals to rustle up when time and money are short, and imaginative ideas for stretching the budget when something more ambitious is called for. The emphasis is on imaginative use of affordable ingredients with the minimum of fuss and equipment.

GRUB ON A GRANT

'. . . a useful little book for the absolute beginner'
Prue Leith, *Guardian*

'. . . full of extremely practical and sensible advice and some hilarious cartoons, giving an exciting repertoire of meals whatever the culinary abilities'
Jill Probert, *Liverpool Daily Post*

NON-FICTION / COOKERY 0 7472 5204 1

A selection of non-fiction from Headline

THE NEXT 500 YEARS	Adrian Berry	£7.99	☐
FIGHTING CANCER	Jonathan Chamberlain	£9.99	☐
LEFT FOOT FORWARD	Garry Nelson	£5.99	☐
THE NATWEST PLAYFAIR CRICKET ANNUAL	Bill Frindall	£4.99	☐
KILLER CULTS	Brian Lane	£6.99	☐
VEGETARIAN GRUB ON A GRANT	Cas Clarke	£5.99	☐
CAPITAL PUNISHMENT	Dougie & Eddy Brimson	£6.99	☐
JUNK FOOD MONKEYS	Robert M Sapolsky	£9.99	☐
PLAYFAIR FOOTBALL WHO'S WHO	Jack Rollin	£6.99	☐
THE TRUTH IN THE LIGHT	Peter and Elizabeth Fenwick	£6.99	☐
THE POLTERGEIST PHENOMENON	John and Anne Spencer	£6.99	☐
MY OLD MAN AND THE SEA	Daniel Hayes and David Hayes	£5.99	☐

All (*Group Division*) books are available at your local bookshop, or can be ordered direct from the publisher. Just tick the titles you would like and complete the details below. Prices and availability are subject to change without prior notice.

Please enclose a cheque or postal order made payable to *Bookpoint Ltd*, and send to: (*Group Division*) 39 Milton Park, Abingdon, OXON, OX14 4TD, UK. Email Address: orders@bookpoint.co.uk

If you would prefer to pay by credit card, our call centre team would be delighted to take your order by telephone. Our direct line *01235 400414* (lines open 9.00 am–6.00 pm Monday to Saturday, 24 hour message answering service). Alternatively you can send a fax on *01235 400454*.

TITLE		FIRST NAME		SURNAME	

ADDRESS	
DAYTIME TEL:		POST CODE	

If you would prefer to pay by credit card, please complete:
Please debit my Visa/Access/Diner's Card/American Express (delete as applicable) card number:

Signature .... Expiry Date ....

If you would *NOT* like to receive further information on our products please tick the box. ☐